I worked as a registered general nurse for 12 years in the NHS. Whilst nursing, I learnt how important nutrition is in helping people in recovery and rehabilitation from illness, disease or surgery.

My nursing experience motivated me to learn more about nutrition and human health. I then went onto study Nutrition and Dietetics at Kings College London University; qualifying as a Registered Dietitian (RD) in 2001. Since then, I have worked in hospitals with people who have diabetes and people with eating disorders. My jobs involved helping people understand how, when and what to eat to improve their health.

At fifty years of age, married with two sons, after thirty years of clinical experience, I now work as a freelance dietitian with a special interest in eating habits and behaviour change.

R. Hutchins

MASTER HEALTHY EATING HABITS

AUSTIN MACAULEY PUBLISHERS™

LONDON * CAMBRIDGE * NEW YORK * SHARJAH

A CIP catalogue record for this title is available from the British Library.

ISBN 9781398440692 (Paperback)
ISBN 9781398440708 (ePub e-book)

www.austinmacauley.com

First Published 2022
Austin Macauley Publishers Ltd®
1 Canada Square
Canary Wharf
London
E14 5AA

A huge thank you to all the hospital staff and patients I have worked with over the last thirty years. Keeping up-to-date with nutrition, physiology and psychology research was not enough to write this book. It was the practical experiences, talking to and working with many different people that made it possible.

Table of Contents

Part 1: How   13

Chapter 1: Motivation   15

Chapter 2: Change Can People Change?   17

Chapter 3: Habits   19

Chapter 4: Meaning and Purpose   29

Chapter 5: Exercise   35

Chapter 6: Support   44

Chapter 7: Body Shape   52

Part 2: When   55

Chapter 8: History   57

Chapter 9: Why Does Fatigue Matter?   61

Chapter 10: How to Control Your Desire for Food (Appetite)   64

Chapter 11: Fasting   75

Chapter 12: Ordered Eating   79

Part 3: What   83

Chapter 13: Foods You Can Swap for a Healthier Alternative   85

Chapter 14: Which Foods are Healthy and Why?   90

Chapter 15: Carbohydrate Foods and the GI   94

Chapter 16: Balanced Diet, Balanced Meals (37)   98

Chapter 17: Vegetables, Salad and Fruit   106

Chapter 18: Protein   109

Chapter 19: Fat   112

Chapter 20: Energy   117

What do I need?   *117*

Chapter 21: Portions   127

How much should I eat? (37, 50, 51)   *127*

Chapter 22: Social Eating   135

Part 4   142

Chapter 23: Main Summary   144

Chapter 24: Health Boosting Changes   150

Chapter 25: Guidelines   154

Chapter 26: What If   158

Chapter 27: References and Further Reading   168

This book is a journey in understanding eating habits and how to make healthy changes that work.

Introduction

Life is a lottery. If people keep themselves slim and active, there is no guarantee they will live a long life free from health problems. **However,** it's widely accepted that choosing to eat healthily and holding a healthy weight puts **the odds in your favour**.

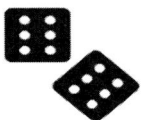

Nowadays, we have unlimited access to online and written advice on how to be healthy and lose weight. Why then, is it difficult to change the way we eat and get fit?

This book is a journey in understanding the **'true picture'** of...

- **HOW** to change eating habits to lose fat and keep it off
- **WHEN** to eat to be in control of your appetite
- **WHAT** to eat to feel more energetic and capable of doing what you want

People can choose from numerous books and online films offering healthy living and exercise advice. There are some inspiring people. Many are popular with millions of views or thousands of books sold. Typically, lifestyle influencers give information on diet, provide recipes and teach people how to exercise. Although each lifestyle or fitness influencer has a different approach, the advice centres on the same basic principles; eat less calories to lose weight, be more active to lose body fat and build muscle. Most of these influencers present themselves as fine examples of health, good looking, well-groomed, athletic body shapes.

Why then aren't we like them?

It is difficult to become like these presenters of health and fitness because they have dramatically changed their lifestyles to become a 'role model'. This demands that they maintain this healthy lifestyle 24/7; it has become their job. The job also earns them a living, hence the books and online views.

Most of us already have a full life with mixed demands of work, family, children, pets, community, running a home, studying, relaxation and entertainment. This doesn't leave much space for dramatic lifestyle change.

The Way I See it is You Have Three Options

1. Continue with your current eating habits and activity. Accept your weight as it is and the fact that over time you will gain more body fat.

2. Try different 'diets' and yoyo from weight loss to weight gain. As you get older, accept gradual loss of muscle and increased body fat.

3. Put effort into understanding and changing your eating and activity habits.
   Lose belly fat, gain muscle.
   Put the odds in your favour for a long life.
   Be fit and capable.
   Feel happier with yourself.
   Be leaner, feel more desirable.

Part 1
How

Chapter 1
Motivation

'A reason or reasons for acting or behaving in a particular way' (1).

Humans have a physical need for nutrition to survive. The human brain drives us to eat, drink and desires food and fluids that taste good. Most of what we consume is chosen because we enjoy it.

The control people have over what food they eat and the activity they do influences their health. The human body can be strong, flexible and capable, if it is cared for. Whatever the state of your body, there are healthy habits that will improve your physical and mental wellbeing.

Dieting is short term
Lifestyle change is long term

Current advice for a 'healthy lifestyle' (2)

1. Drink more water and less alcohol
2. Eat more foods high in fibre
3. Do not ban food, swap for a healthier alternative
4. Add more fruit and vegetables into your meals
5. Eat regular meals with structured snacks
6. Find a simple way of being more active

Sounds straight forward, so why then is it difficult to consistently behave this way?

Health education gives people knowledge but doesn't always change behaviour. Knowing we should choose healthy foods and take regular exercise does not necessarily make us do it (3).

During my 30 years working as a nurse and then as a dietitian, I observed that people do not follow diets planned by someone else for very long. What works is helping people to decide for themselves what they are willing or able to change.

- Do you want to lose body fat?
- Do you want to improve your physical and mental health?

If you answered yes to these questions, then you are motivated.

Chapter 2
Change Can People Change?

Change depends on a person's life experience and circumstances. Basically, the demands of work and family will influence when you eat and how much. You may have tried to lose weight in the past but then lapsed back into old eating habits.

What was going on in your life that made it difficult to change the way you ate and cared for yourself?

Being 'healthy' means changing habits that we do every day without thinking.

The longer you have been repeating the same eating habits, the more effort and time it will take to change them.

Do you want to change?

We are more likely to resist change if our unhealthy habits give us something we need. People drink alcohol and smoke cigarettes because it makes them feel good and helps us deal with life's difficulties. Eating food is a great pleasure and an important part of work, family and social life.

Do you want to improve your health by changing how, when and what you eat?

Is losing body fat and getting fit as important as other demands in your life?

If you answered yes, then you are ready to change.

Summary – motivation and change

- ❖ People feel good if they eat food and drink, they enjoy.
- ❖ Is losing weight as important as other significant parts of your life, such as, family, work, entertainment, hobbies, socialising, relaxation and rest?
- ❖ Choosing to eat healthy foods and increasing activity may improve quality of life, physical and mental health and extend lives (4, 5, 6, 7).
- ❖ Old eating and activity habits have caused weight gain and current habits make it difficult to lose.

Chapter 3
Habits

Habit – 'usual way of behaving or tendency someone has settled into' (1).

Habits are important

Habits shape our life more than we realise.

Habits are strong and happen spontaneously (without thinking).

Habits create brain cravings (neurological). A brain craving is strong urge to do something. People can experience mental discomfort if they are not able to eat or drink what they want.

Humans are driven to keep repeating the same behaviour because we are rewarded by the release of 'pleasure chemicals' in the brain.

- It takes a minimum of three months of planning, preparing and repeating a new way of eating to create a new habit.
- Over time, these choices become an action that you do without thinking.
- These actions become established habits and the habits become a way of life.

45% of behaviours are repeated everyday.

These are your habits. Most of the time we repeat habits like choosing the food we want to eat or drinking alcohol without questioning whether we should change it.

Why do we keep repeating the same behaviours even if it is bad for our health?

The human brain seeks to minimise effort so behaviours that you repeat everyday become automatic. If you do something without much thought, it is a lot easier for the brain and body to cope because it involves less effort.

To be able to change unhealthy habits it helps if you understand how habits form (8, 9).

Eating habits happen like this

1. **Trigger** – a signal that prompts you to an action such as eating or drinking.

   Feeling thirsty or tired or hungry or in a low mood are all triggers. Just the sight of food or drinks can be enough to make people want to eat.

   Another trigger would be someone offering to share food which is accepted even if a person does not feel hungry.

Triggers that happens outside of your body (external)

- Sight or smell of food
- Watching others eat
- Advertisements or watching cooking programmes
- Planned or unplanned demands from our work or private life which make us feel stressed

External triggers are more likely to make us eat when we have no physical triggers (internal) that remind us to eat.

Physical sensations from within the human body that signal we are hungry (internal triggers)

- Empty stomach that growls and gurgles
- Headache
- Lightheaded feeling
- Grumpy and less tolerant

- Lack of energy
- Shakiness and general feeling of weakness

2. **Routine** – a habit that doesn't vary. Happens every day. It may be that work, or home environments have food and drinks nearby. People see food and eat it or want to eat the same as others to 'fit in'. Eating whatever food is available or meal served, especially if they were not involved in planning or preparation.

3. **Reward** – Eating food or drinking alcohol gives people something, makes us feel 'good' or relaxed or relieved. Helps deal with 'feeling' bad, sad, unhappy or tired.

4. *Whenever there is a trigger and the urge to get the reward, we will repeat the same habit.*

Examples

 On the way home from work, a person starts thinking about drinking a glass of wine or having a beer when they get home. This is using alcohol to 'unwind' in the evening.

If a person has been busy all day and not had time to eat much food, they will eat an evening meal, then keep snacking, because they are hungry, tired and have not eaten enough earlier in the day.

5 Healthy habits recommended by the UK NHS 2018 (2)

1. Not smoking
2. Eat a healthy diet
3. Regular exercise – 30 to 60 minutes a day of moderate to vigorous activity (makes you feel hot, sweat, increases heart rate).

4. Keeping a healthy body weight (BMI 18.5–24.9)
5. Moderate alcohol consumption

Recommended no more than 14 units in a week or 2 units every day.
1 unit = ½ pint beer/lager/bitter (around 4% ABV) OR 175ml wine or single shot spirits 25ml.

How do I change?
Think about…
What are my triggers?

Tick the box that is the nearest reflection of your current lifestyle

When do you eat?

Meals and snacks		Tick box
I eat breakfast*	Most days	✓
	Sometimes	
	Never	
I eat a 'lighter' or 'snack' meal* *(lunch or midday meal)* *(small cooked meal or sandwich)*	Every day	✓
	Sometimes	
	Never	
I snack between my meals*	In the morning	
	In the afternoon	✓
	I snack in the evening	✓
I eat an evening meal* **(dinner or supper)** *(main cooked meal of the day)*	Every day	✓
	Sometimes	
	Never	

A meal is an occasion when people sit down and eat, usually at a regular time.

How much do you eat?

Snacks		Tick box
If I want to snack, I would choose to eat one food snack or have a drink that contains calories (*fruit juice, smoothie or latte or hot chocolate or sugary fizzy drink, cappuccino*)	Most days	✓
	Sometimes	
	Never	
If I eat one snack, I would end up eating several	Most days	✓
	Sometimes	
	Never	

Meals		Tick box
I do not prepare meals*; I eat what I am served	Most days	
	Sometimes	✓
	Never	
Majority of the meals* I eat are readymade or takeaways	Most days	
	Sometimes	✓
	Never	
My main meal *of the day fills a meal plate	Most days	✓
	Sometimes	
	Never	
My main meal *of the day fills a meal plate and I have a second helping	Most days	
	Sometimes	✓
My main meal* of the day fills a meal plate and I eat a dessert or snack after the meal	Most days	✓
	Sometimes	
	Never	

A main meal usually takes more time to prepare and involves combining different foods that are cooked, mixed or served together; one to three courses. A 'light' or snack meal is smaller, readymade or quick to prepare. Some people serve the main meal at midday, with supper as the late afternoon/early evening meal, while others may call their midday meal lunch and their early evening meal supper or dinner.

When do you drink alcohol?

Alcohol		Tick box
When do you drink alcohol	Every day	
	Most evenings	
	Once or twice a week	
	Never	✓

When are you active?

		Tick box
I will spend at least one-hour walking	Every day	
	Most days	
	Once or twice a week	✓
	Rarely	
I exercise or play a sport	Every day	
	Most days	
	Once or twice a week	✓
	Rarely	

These questions help show the reality of your current eating and activity habits.

As you continue reading this book your answers to these questions will be useful in planning what you want to change.

The brain is 'programmed' by human history
to do whatever it takes to survive

Humans have survived over thousands of years because people
'see food, eat food'
Food makes us feel good and gives us energy to think clearly and move around.

This is…

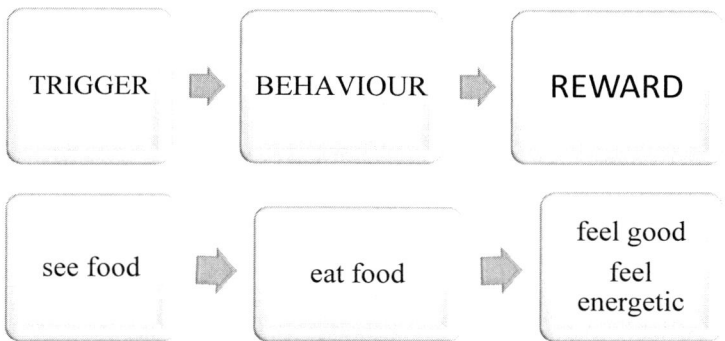

We repeat this; it becomes impulsive to repeat this
behaviour whenever there is a trigger (10)

It becomes a habit when you are no longer aware of the trigger and do the unhealthy behaviour without thinking (11).

Changing habits takes planning
The process is…

THOUGHT

- Plan what you want to change.
- *Example, desire to lose belly fat and eat a healthy diet.*

EFFORT

- Put changes into action.
- Gain experience in choosing healthy foods, controlling meal portions and becoming more active.

RESIST URGES

- Human brains are comfortable with old patterns of behaviour.
- The brain thinks change is dangerous and disruptive to survival.
- Your brain will want to return to old behaviours.

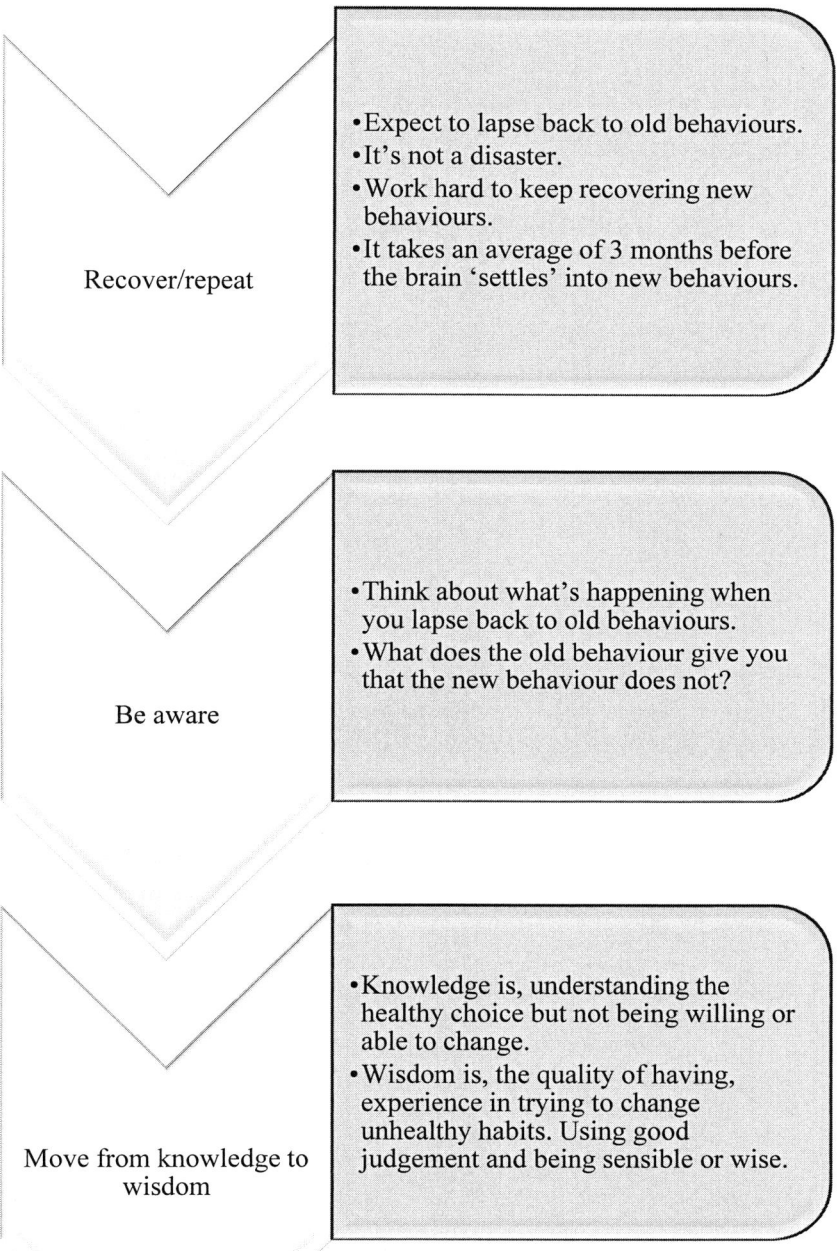

Recover/repeat

- Expect to lapse back to old behaviours.
- It's not a disaster.
- Work hard to keep recovering new behaviours.
- It takes an average of 3 months before the brain 'settles' into new behaviours.

Be aware

- Think about what's happening when you lapse back to old behaviours.
- What does the old behaviour give you that the new behaviour does not?

Move from knowledge to wisdom

- Knowledge is, understanding the healthy choice but not being willing or able to change.
- Wisdom is, the quality of having, experience in trying to change unhealthy habits. Using good judgement and being sensible or wise.

Consider the **positive traits in your personality** that will help you change established habits.

Examples:

If you like to write lists, keep appointments or schedule your day use these skills to start planning what you will eat and when each day. This brings order into eating and a sense of control over your own body.

Exercise is a great replacement for alcohol or overeating because it releases endorphins. Endorphins are natural chemicals released by your brain that make you feel good. They lift your mood by making you feel more positive and confident. Plus, being more active burns more calories and changes the composition of your body to more muscle and less body fat.

Summary – Habits

- ❖ When people see food, they may not feel hungry but end up eating because they like the taste or want to 'fit in' with other people.
- ❖ Think about eating habits that happen every day. The times that you eat, times that you are active, times that you drink alcohol. All humans have patterns of behaviour that are repeated.
- ❖ **Change is possible when people understand the reality of their behaviour and plan what to do differently**.

Chapter 4

Meaning and Purpose

Purpose – 'The reason for which something is done. A person's sense of determination' (1).

People try to lose weight by restricting what they eat and exercising, only to give up the exercise and return to old eating habits. **These changes would have been competing against years of established eating and activity habits.**

If people want to change their eating habits it helps if the new healthy behaviours are supporting something they care about. This gives '**meaning and purpose**' to changing the way a person eats rather than being on a 'diet'.

What do you care about?

- Have you gained body fat and feel certain that you want to lose it?
- Do you remember what you looked like when you were slimmer?
- Are some of your clothes too small? Want to wear them again?
- Have you been diagnosed with a health problem that would improve if you lost weight?
- Do you know someone who has health problems or someone who died? Has this motivated you to take better care of yourself?
- Do you care about the environment and climate change and want to change the food you buy and the way you travel to help prevent global warming?
- Do you care for animals and are against cruelty so would value being a vegetarian or vegan?
- Do you want to live a long life and have quality of life?

Quality of life means a state of physical, mental and social well-being. No disease or physical or mental problems that limit the way you want to live.

- Does religion or faith give spiritual guidance to care for yourself as much as you would care for others?

 Benefits of being a healthy weight (2)

Health Benefits   *Personal Benefits*

Reduces High Blood Pressure   More energy

Improves Cholesterol levels   Fit into smaller clothes, so more choice

Reduces risk of type 2 diabetes   Movement takes less effort. Able to be more active with your family and exercise is easier

Improves control of blood glucose levels if you have type 2 diabetes   Feel fitter

Lowers risk of death from cancer, diabetes or heart disease   Sleep improves

Improves lung function in asthma   Don't feel so hot, sweat less

                                     More likely to live longer

Reduces osteoarthritis (loss of Breathing is easier
cartilage around knee and hip joints)

More stable blood
glucose levels

Psychological benefits of being a healthy weight (2)

Increased self-esteem

Reduction in depressive symptoms

Improved body image

Improved quality of life

More likely to socialise

Lower levels of anxiety

Physically capable of being more active so can
gain the psychological benefits of exercise
Releases natural feel good hormones endorphins

Reminder of Healthy Habits (2)

1. Eat lots of fruit and vegetables. 5 to 8 portions a day.
2. Don't smoke or give up for at least 5 years.
3. Regular exercise – 5 to 7 hours a week.
4. Drink in moderation – 1 to 3 units a day. Limit to 14 units in a week.
5. If you are overweight BMI 25–29.9. If you do all of 1 to 4 healthy habits, you will be at lower risk of early death. The same as people who are a healthy weight BMI 18.5 to 24.9.

What is a healthy weight?

Weight or clothes size does not take into account a person's height. So, weight is usually converted to body mass index or BMI; **weight (in kgs)/height (m^2)**

Standard World Health Organisation classifications for BMI (12)

BMI

Healthy weight	18.5–24.99
Overweight	25–29.99
Obese	30–39.99
Morbidly Obese	40 and over

A better way of judging how much body fat you have is from your waist measurement.

Knowing your BMI is helpful, but waist measurements of more than 40 inches or 102 cm for men and 34.5 inches or 88 cm for women put people at risk of serious health conditions. Research has linked too much 'belly' fat with a greater risk of developing heart disease, high blood pressure, stroke, cancer and type 2 diabetes (12).

To measure your waist, feel the bottom of your ribs and the top of your hips. In the middle of these two points wrap a tape measure around, breathe out naturally, relax, then take the measurement.

UK recommendations

It doesn't matter what clothing size people fit into or how tall they are, it is beneficial to health to lose belly fat to measure…

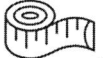
Less than 37 inches or **94 cm** for men

Less than 31.5 inches or **80 cm** for women

Guidelines for people of Black African, Middle Eastern, White European and mixed origin.

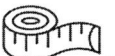
Less than 35.4 inches or **90 cm** for Men

Less than 31.5 inches or **80 cm** for Women

Recommended healthy waist measurement for people from African Caribbean, South Asian, Chinese and Japanese origins.

African Caribbean, South Asian, Chinese and Japanese people tend to carry more fat and less muscle, so the risk of diabetes, heart and circulatory diseases starts to increase at a lower weight than for Black African, White European, Middle Eastern and Mixed origin people.

Top 5 causes of premature* death UK (13) | **Unhealthy Habits most likely to cause disease**

1. *Cancer* — Smoking

2. *Ischaemic heart Disease and stroke*

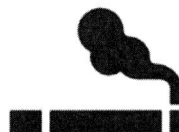

33

3. *Lung Disease – Influenza, pneumonia, chronic lower respiratory diseases*

4. *Liver disease – alcoholism or fatty liver*   Alcohol and/or obesity

5. *Dementia and Alzheimer's disease*

*Premature is dying before the average age of death in a population.
In 2019, England life expectancy in years – Males = 79.9, Females = 83.6

Health brings a freedom very few realise,
until they no longer have it

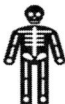 **You have one life one body**

Summary – Meaning and purpose

❖ Choosing a lifestyle that strongly supports eating healthy foods and being more active gives a 'clear' reason and purpose to stick to new habits.

❖ Other people are more likely to support you with healthy behaviour changes because they can identify with the purpose and meaning of your lifestyle.

❖ If your purpose is to be healthy because of a physical or mental problem, recent bereavement or as part of caring for animals or the environment, you will be more determined to avoid unhealthy food choices.

Chapter 5
Exercise

'Activity that requires physical effort, carried out to sustain or improve health and fitness' (1).

How exercising helps your body (14)

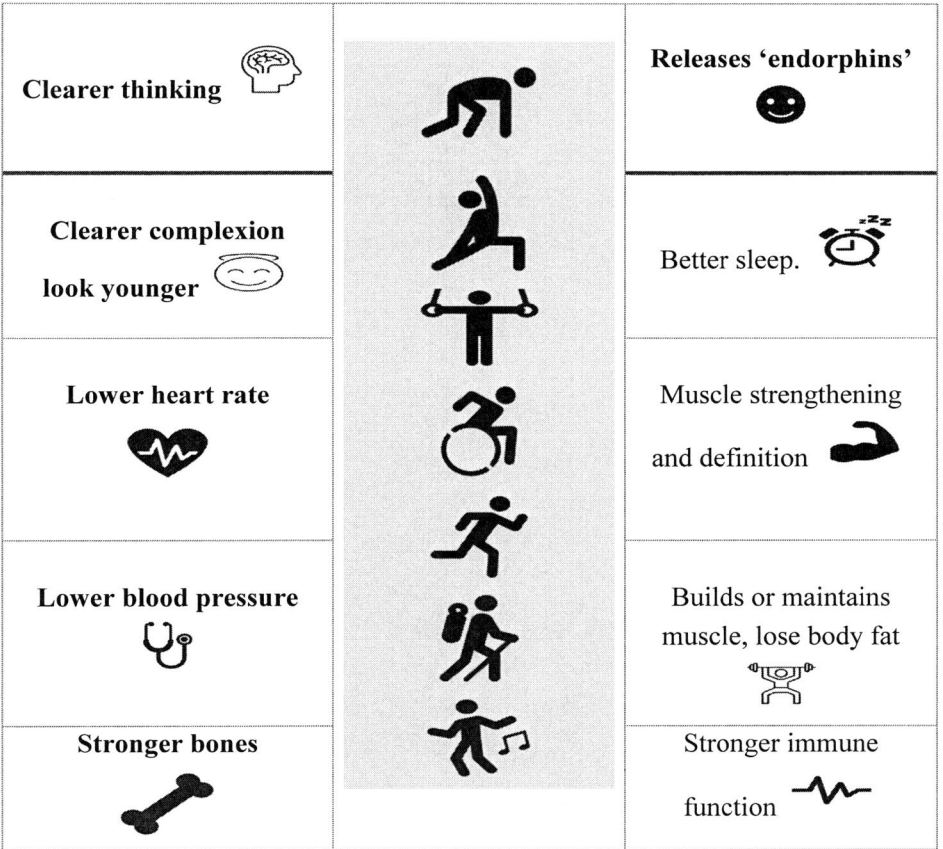

Muscles support joints better 		

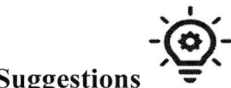

Think about your lifestyle

On a typical weekday and a day at the weekend.

- ❖ How much time would you spend on your feet moving around?
- ❖ How much time do you spend sitting?
- ❖ How much time do you spend sleeping?

Add it up in rough hours.

There are 24 hours in a day. Start planning how **one** of these hours could be dedicated to exercise.

If you are thinking I cannot fit exercise in, I am too busy in the day and too tired by the evening, look at the reality of how you spend your time. It's unlikely you can add in an hour of exercise because you do not believe you have free time. Think about whether you could swap or drop something out to exercise? Could you combine socialising with exercise; going for a walk or bicycle ride or attend an exercise class with your partner, friend or family.

Suggestions

Consider swapping 1 hour of screen time, TV, Netflix, phones, iPad/tablets, laptops, computers **for exercise**.

If you work long hours, 10–14 hours a days, could you build activity into your day by walking to or from work? Could you get up earlier and do an **exercise routine before work or the school run?**

What about **joining a gym, could you do a class before you go to work**. If your job is mentally demanding, exercising early morning before work is reported to **lower 'stress' hormones (adrenaline and cortisol)** during your workday. This helps to prevent some of the aging and weight gain effects of a demanding work life. Workers who go to the gym are said to be 'burning off the adrenaline'.

Which exercise?

Yoga, Pilates or body balance would suit people who have physically demanding jobs, where people are on their feet most of the day, having to move around a lot or any jobs that involve lifting.

A Yoga session is mainly muscular exercise. It also calms the part of your brain that makes humans feel anxiety, so would suit people who feel mentally and physically drained at the end of a workday, such as carers, nurses, doctors or mental health workers.

Yoga involves deep breathing with muscular movement. It would be beneficial for people who have difficulty breathing (asthma, COPD, smokers).

If your job involves sitting down most of the day, any regular activity that gets you moving and raises your heart rate will improve your health.

Do you find it difficult to self-motivate? Look at exercise classes in your area. Start going with a friend or partner to build your confidence and to establish exercise as a routine part of your lifestyle.

What if you hate exercise?

 What do you hate?

- ❖ Getting out of breath or feeling tired quickly?
- ❖ Does your heart rate feel too fast?
- ❖ Do you dislike getting hot and sweating?
- ❖ Feel uncomfortable in 'gym gear'?
- ❖ Do not like exercising surrounded by other fit people?

These are problems of being overweight and unfit. All of these problems will be solved if you commit to being more active and lose excess body fat.

The human body is brilliant at adapting to exercise. A person's fitness level will improve within a month if they exercise at least 3 to 4 times a week.

If you don't want to join a gym or do any sports, then be more active whenever you can and do not set yourself goals that you cannot stick to because it may give you a sense of failure. Any increase in activity is better than being inactive. Maybe start by walking every day or exercising at home.

The trouble with losing fat is when people decide 'I want to lose weight', they want fast results. This is more likely to drive people to severe food restriction with bursts of exercise that only last for a few weeks.

In the UK, there are almost 10 million gym members. So, one out or every seven people has a gym membership.

Anyone who has been a member of a gym for a while knows it is very busy from New Year to about March then attendance starts to decline, by June half the people who exercised in January no longer attend; there are reasons for this (see history section).

Plan exercise when you are most likely to do it
What happens to the human body with regular exercise (15)?

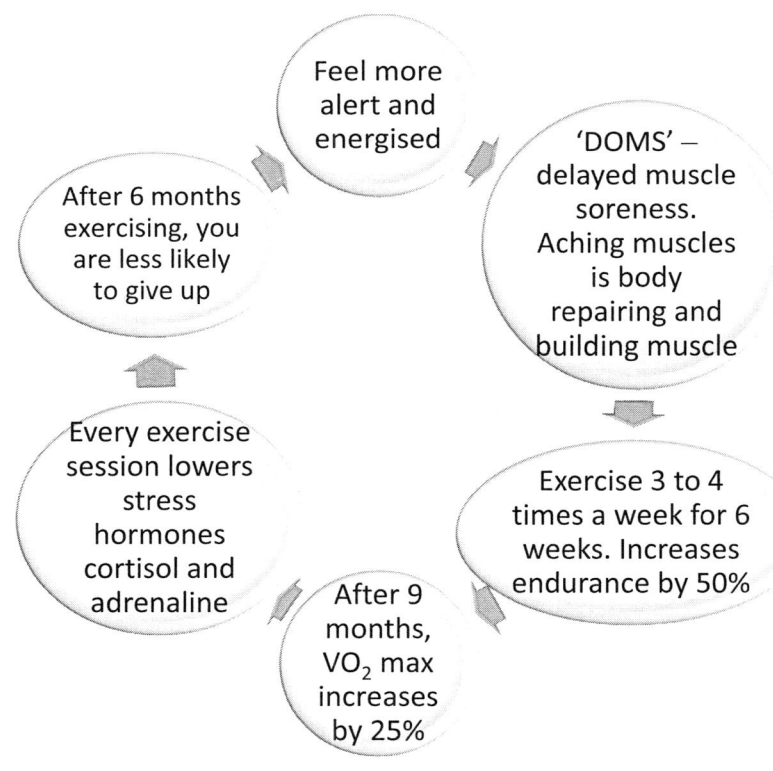

Feel more alert and energised

'DOMS' – delayed muscle soreness. Aching muscles is body repairing and building muscle

After 6 months exercising, you are less likely to give up

Every exercise session lowers stress hormones cortisol and adrenaline

After 9 months, VO$_2$ max increases by 25%

Exercise 3 to 4 times a week for 6 weeks. Increases endurance by 50%

- ➢ **VO₂ max** is the speed your body transports oxygen. Increasing your VO_2 max means you can exercise more intensely for longer.
- ➢ We '**burn off**' the stress hormones **cortisol and adrenaline** with exercise. This reduces feelings of anxiety and depression during the day particularly if you can exercise first thing in the morning.

UK Chief Medical Officers 2019 (17)
Guidelines for adult exercise each week are:

Recommends **2 ½ hours of moderate intensity** exercise *(breathing and heart rate increase, feel warmer, can still hold a conversation)* such as brisk walking.

PLUS **1 ¼ hours of high intensity exercise** (*high heart rate, feel hot, sweating, breathing more rapid, difficult to hold conversation*).

AS WELL AS **2 days of workouts that strengthen and condition muscles**; weight training, callisthenics, yoga, Pilates.

US Department of Health (16)

150 minutes or 2 ½ hours of moderate intensity exercise

PLUS 75 minutes or 1 ¼ hours of vigorous activity

AS WELL AS strengthening activity, muscular exercises on two days a week

As you can see, it is the same recommendations in the UK as it is in America.

This is 6 hours of activity in a week. Depending on how you fit the 6 hours of exercise into your life; plan at least one muscle rest day.

Exercise on its own does not result in much weight loss

Exercise changes the composition of the human body. This means we gain muscle and lose fat, which is much better for your health. The weighing scales may not show much actual loss, but your clothes will be looser as muscle is dense so holds a tighter firmer body shape. Plus, muscles are 'calorie burning' cells so as you gain muscle, you will use up more calories more efficiently through the whole day.

Humans have evolved a large brain that is adaptable and can coordinate complex movements

There is a powerful connection between the health of your brain and movement. It has been reported that regular exercise primes your brain to learn faster (20).

Exercise increases dopamine storage

Dopamine is a 'feel good' hormone. Higher levels have been associated with increased motivation and focus. When dopamine and serotonin levels are low, we feel depressed.

It is widely recognised that exercisers feel less depressed (21).

Have a look at the exercises listed, see which would suit you. If you stick to just one or two types of exercise, the ability to change your body shape will be limited. Human bodies quickly adapt to any physical demands put on them. So, we need to **'mix up'** exercise to challenge different muscles. This works better to develop an athletic body shape.

If people train a lot in one particular exercise, their body adapts, and the muscles are shaped to be able to do those movements well.

Examples:

> Marathon runners keep skinny and light because it's easier to run fast for a long distance if you don't weigh much.

> Rugby players, wrestlers and weightlifters are large, muscly and powerful because they have to grapple with other large, muscly people or lift heavy weights to compete in their sport.

> Swimmers have a strong all-round muscly shape because they have to move their body weight against the resistance of water.

> Cyclists have large, powerful, leg muscles with weak upper bodies because all the energy to drive the bike is from the legs.

➤ Yoga or Pilates is a mainly muscular exercise that works the whole body. Because it involves a lot of stretching, muscles are strong and flexible so look toned without building bulk.

Consider doing a mixture of these exercises

Exercise	Benefits to body	Rate of calorie burning
Walking	• Heart and lungs (cardiovascular) • Endurance • Works leg muscles	*Moderate during walking*
Jogging or running	• Heart and lungs • (cardiovascular) • Endurance • Works most muscles	*Fast whilst running or jogging*
Cycling	• Heart and lungs • (cardiovascular) • Endurance • Works leg muscles	*Fast whilst cycling*
Weight training	• Muscle building • Strength	*Burns calories less intensely than cardiovascular exercise THEN increases calories used by body over the whole day*
Interval training – *short bursts of high intensity exercise*	• Heart and lungs • Muscle strength and endurance	
Swimming	• Heart and lungs • Muscle strength and endurance	

| **Yoga, Pilates, Body Balance or Tai Chi** | • Muscle strength and flexibility
• Mentally calming |

Cardiovascular exercise is aerobic

Aerobic means it uses up calories and oxygen quickly. So, cycling or running would make our heart rate increase and breathing more rapid to get more oxygen into the bloodstream.

Muscular or anaerobic exercise

Involves short bursts of intense muscle movements; lifting your own body weight as in yoga or lifting heavy weights in weightlifting. **Anaerobic exercise** burns less calories during the activity when compared to **aerobic activity** (running, cycling). After anaerobic activity, the body burns more calories when you are resting.

Duke University (18) completed a study where they asked 119 people who were overweight to do either cardiovascular exercise or weight training or a mix of both.

This is what they found...

The people who did aerobic training lost weight. The weight change was measured and found to be a mix of fat, water and muscle tissue.

People who only did weight training with no aerobic exercise gained weight. This was measured and reported as a gain of 2 lb of muscle.

The people who did both weight training and cardiovascular exercise showed the best improvements. They lost weight, maintained muscle mass and lost belly fat (reduced waist circumference).

The **Duke University study recommended** doing weight training first and then cardiovascular exercise. The weight training drops your stores of glucose so your body switches to use more fat for energy during cardiovascular exercise.

Summary – Exercise

➢ Exercise **positively improves** a person's physical and mental health.

➢ Think about where exercise will fit into your day. **Exercise that can be included in everyday life will have the biggest 'calorie' burning impact** on your body.

➢ **Any increase in activity is better than doing no exercise**. If you are unfit, start with an activity you can do, like walking or exercise at home in private. This will improve your cardiovascular fitness (heart and lungs) and build your confidence to try other exercise or play sports.

Chapter 6
Support

To support someone simply means that you offer to help them. This works best if support is mutual.

During my years working as a dietitian, people would describe how meals and snacks were fitted in around the demands of their day. Food was not always a priority compared to all the other things they needed to do. They relied on ready-made foods, takeaways or left the responsibility of food shopping, meal planning and preparation to a partner or other family.

Part of my job as a dietitian would be to ask people to give me an idea of when they ate, what they ate and who prepared the food. People would have similar themes; these are a few examples:

- o If a person had a partner, typically one person would take on the main responsibility for planning, preparing and serving their food. The person who did not have lead responsibility for planning and preparing meals would be more likely to eat what they were given.
- o Few people would have an idea of roughly the calories their body needed or know how many calories were in the foods they ate the most often.
- o People found it easier if foods were identified as either good or bad. The old promotion of healthy eating, to eat everything in moderation meant nothing to individuals. It doesn't tell people how much should go on their plate or what foods to eat.
- o Some people do not like healthy eating, believing lower calorie meals to be tasteless. Numerous individuals don't like eating vegetables or salad. Plus, healthy eating is presented on television or online as requiring the time and skills to cook from raw ingredients whilst following a recipe. A large proportion of people are not interested in this, they do not feel

they have the time, and just want to know what to eat when they feel hungry.

- o If individuals who wanted to lose weight ate less in a day or missed meals, they would consider themselves as having been 'good'. People would be less likely to maintain their 'diet' if they ate out or went on a holiday. A common comment would be something like 'I don't worry about what I eat on a holiday'. Eating out at a restaurant or friend's house would be permission to indulge in eating large meals or several courses not leaving any food because 'I've paid for it' or 'It's rude to leave food that a friend or family has made for you'. These kinds of behaviours trap people into a cycle of 'dieting or being good', which then 'justifies' or gives them permission to indulge in random episodes of overeating.

Think for a minute about these habits, do they encourage disordered eating and a sense of whatever I do, I can't lose weight. Are random episodes of social or holiday overeating really excessive indulgence or binge eating?

If you want to lose weight and keep it off, changes to your eating habits need to be continued when you eat out, when other people provide food for you and on holidays.

So far, we have established it's hard to change eating habits and it takes a lot of planning, motivation and effort to change your lifestyle, but **it's not impossible**.

Nobody likes to be told they are overweight or obese

People who are overweight know they are fat and do not want someone pointing it out.

Speak to the people you eat with on a regular basis

Let them know you are trying to change the way you eat. It is helpful to aim for a healthier lifestyle rather than being on a diet. If your goal is to lose weight quickly for an event, such as a wedding or holiday, you will need to dramatically reduce calories eaten and exercise. The problem with short-term episodes of extreme dieting and exercise is that these new behaviours are less likely to be maintained long term because your brain has spent many years repeating old eating patterns and it will end up driving you to recover the weight you lost.

The human brain does better with small changes that are repeated over a long time. **'Repeating an ordered meal pattern'** allows the human brain to adapt to these new eating behaviours. As the months pass, these new healthy behaviours become the normal.

Food is great it's one of life's pleasures

We get to enjoy eating meals two or three times a day. Nevertheless, food is just energy and nutrients for body function. We can enjoy eating meals, desserts, snacks and be in control.

An incredibly positive step to being healthy and losing body fat is to commit to taking full responsibility for all the food you eat.

It helps to be in control by planning and serving all your meals and snacks.

You do not have to prepare all your food or cook but should **take charge of what goes on the plate**. Be aware of what you eat and start having a look at how many calories are in the foods you eat the most often.

If you eat out, commit to eating only two courses

Be determined. Don't allow yourself to be pressured into extras or second helpings or another pint or glass of wine. What helps is if you plan in your head what you will eat and drink before you go out.

Alcohol will loosen inhibitions so you would be more likely to eat, or drink more than you planned. If other people are being indulgent, they are likely to want others to join in. Some people feel uncomfortable in a group if they are the only one drinking alcohol or eating a dessert. They may try to persuade others to eat and drink as much as them.

Be clear with yourself what you are going to eat or drink before you go. It helps if you divert responsibility to someone else, such as, my doctor or dietitian told me I need to change/follow this diet. Most people would not pressure someone to eat or drink alcohol if they know it would be bad for their health.

Partners or family can find it hard if you want to change the way you eat.

They may resist letting go of the control, they have over planning, shopping, preparing and serving your meals. It could be a combination of habit, cooking a lot of food and serving large portions. Providing food and being generous is strongly connected to caring for someone. If a partner, friend or family puts effort into preparing meals, they could feel offended if you do not want to eat all the food offered. Sometimes both partners may be overweight and only one of them wants to change eating habits.

It's normal for a different routine to be resisted by the human brain so you would be wise to discuss the alterations to your eating with your partner, friends or family away from the mealtime. If you can agree to make 'healthy changes' together, it's more likely to continue long term.

Have a look at the guidelines written below

Consider sharing these points with people who eat meals with you on a regular basis.

➢ Be a cheerleader, not a coach. Offer encouragement rather than telling others what to do.
➢ No one changes eating and exercise and maintains those changes perfectly.
➢ Talk about it, but away from any eating or mealtime. Anxiety or feelings of deprivation are highest at mealtimes. If habits are discussed while you are eating, it's much more likely to stir up resentment and end in an argument.
➢ Listen to each other; keep judgement in your head.
➢ **Best line ever**, '*Is there anything I can do to help you?*'
➢ If you don't feel able to offer positive encouragement, it's best if you don't say anything, just listen.

It is common for dietitians to be sent referrals of overweight or obese people from other health professionals such as GPs. The referral is made by a doctor because in their professional opinion losing body fat would improve this person's health. If the patient did not think there was anything wrong with the foods they ate, they may be resistant or contemptuous of dietary change. Some individuals would put up barriers or sabotage discussion with the dietitian. For example, most people would give you an account of what they typically ate on a 'good' day or 'diet' day. I would discuss changes to their eating that would help, which would be blocked by comments 'I tried that it didn't work', or 'I didn't lose weight'. Others would not see how what they ate could change because someone else did the food shopping and prepared meals. Some denied ever snacking, which is unlikely especially if you consider the liquid calories that go in hot drinks with milk, fruit juice drinks or biscuits with a tea or coffee.

The point of this is **not** to moan about people trying to lose weight. It's to emphasise that no dietary advice is any help if you do not feel ready or willing to change the way you eat.

 Knowing what you should eat and what you should avoid does not necessarily make you do it.

People crave the 'pleasure' hit from eating sweet and fatty foods. The drive to eat is your brain chasing that feeling. This powerful dopamine lift only lasts with the first few mouthfuls of food or the first 1 to 2 units of alcohol. After that, it's downhill; you're either left feeling guilty about the amount of food you just ate or getting drunk.

Your past eating and activity habits have made you overweight, and your current habits prevent weight loss.

Individuals can only lose body fat if they are willing to change their eating, drinking and activity behaviours. Otherwise, overweight or obese people will stay the same weight and are more likely to gradually get fatter as they age.

The most important step to a healthier lifestyle with a leaner body is too take full responsibility for everything you choose to eat and drink.

Have a look at these stages of change (22, 23)

Can you relate to any of the behaviours in these stages?

You may not be in one spot, more likely to be moving backwards and forwards over 2 or 3.

Pre-contemplation 'No not me'	Contemplation 'Well maybe'	Determination / Preparation Okay, so what do I do now?	Action 'Okay, let's do this'	Maintenance 'It is possible'
Eats what you want when you want	Becomes aware of the negative effects of being overweight	Wants to lose body fat Understands pattern or triggers, behaviour and reward	Uses meal plan or food diary to set up daily food intake	Able to choose foods because they are healthy
Eats when feeling emotional or is *triggered Gains pleasure from food and feels better whilst eating	Interested in the personal benefit of losing fat Got some idea of the changes that need to be made	Establishes ways to change old habits Creates a meal plan to use as a strategy	Journals thoughts and feelings that occur around mealtimes	Plans and serves balanced meals and enjoys the taste
Keeps eating beyond feeling 'full'. Stops at 'Stuffed'	Feels uncertain how to cope with feeling hungry	Identifies interfering behaviours that 'trigger' old eating habits Anticipates and prepares for challenges and triggers	Starts to include 'healthier' food choices Plans controlled social eating	Able to ignore 'hunger pangs' between meals and planned snacks Knows when and where to nourish herself/himself healthily
Eats snacks and leftovers, nibbles at food when alone or in secret	Begins to consider what it would be like to eat less, eat healthily and exercise	Speaks to people who are willing to help and asks for their support	Asks for help and support from family and friends	Feels comfortable eating in a controlled manner in social settings
Thoughts are preoccupied by food. Feel				

49

strong urges to eat	Keeps structured mealtimes	Able to maintain meal and snack
Fears not having food available to eat	Starts recognising and 'sitting with' and not acting on the drive to eat more. Practices 'surfing' the urge to eat.	routine that meets their energy needs Requests support when needed

Relapse
'Here we go again'

- **Can occur at any of the stages**
- **People may find themselves moving backwards and forwards through the different stages**
- **Cycle of change may need to be repeated several times on the journey to healthier eating habits**
- **Understanding your triggers to overeating and how you can change these behaviours means you will move yourself out of pre-contemplation and contemplation quicker.**
- **Recognise the stage you are at, plan how to move forward and ask for support.**

*Trigger feelings – Happiness, sexual frustration, fear, anxiety, 'bad' day, tired, lonely, low mood, depressed, eating as part of entertainment and socialising (watching TV, films, takeaways, restaurants).

Summary – Support

- It is important to think about 'do you feel ready or able to change eating and activity habits?'
- Discuss the changes you want to make to your eating and activity with partners or significant people who you eat meals with.
- Each time you try to change eating habits, you will learn what works and what does not. Lapses back to old habits are not a failure; problem solve what went wrong and try again.
- You are responsible for everything you eat and drink.

Chapter 7
Body Shape

Which genetic body shape is most like you? (24)

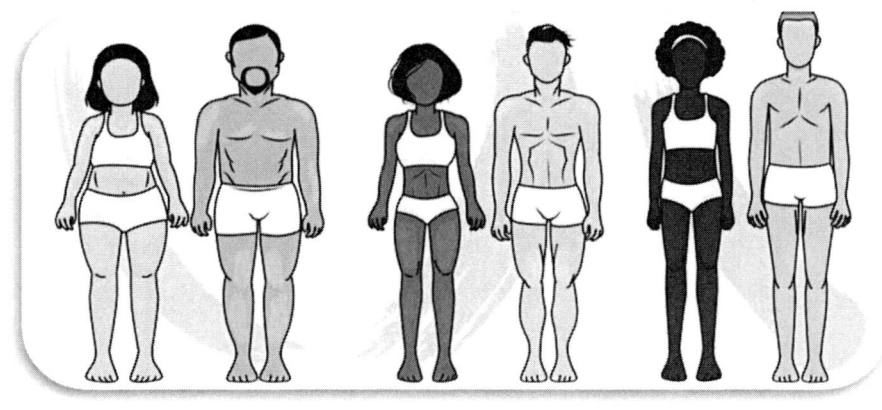

Endomorph	Mesomorph	Ectomorph

Endomorph

Build is stocky with thick legs and arms and a rounder body. Thick rib cage with hips as wide as the shoulders. Naturally muscly and strong. Can gain muscle easily but can also gain fat. If Endomorphs become overweight, fat will build up under the skin over most of their body not just around the abdomen (belly fat).

Mesomorph

Body shape is rectangular with wide shoulders and a narrow waist.

Naturally have a muscly build and are able to do any exercise or sports. They can lose or gain weight depending on how much they eat and how active they are. If Mesomorphs becomes overweight, they put fat on mainly around the abdomen (belly fat).

Ectomorph

Build is tall with narrow shoulders and hips. Long arms and legs. Ectomorphs suit cardiovascular exercise such as running or athletics where it is an advantage to have a body shape that is thin and light. If Ectomorphs become overweight, they will put fat on mainly around the abdomen (belly fat).

You can't change your genetic body shape. Some physical characteristics such as your height, bone structure, size of your feet and hands, eye colour, places you carry excess body fat cannot be changed.

It is a massive help if people can accept their genetic body shape and focus on taking better care of themselves.

Taking good care of your body will always benefit your physical and mental health.

How does the shape of the human body change if we lose fat and build muscle?

An athletic body shape or looking 'fit' is defined by its muscle mass. Muscles that are kept active have a firm 'toned' appearance. Only muscle gives good body shape. Body fat is 'spare' stored energy under the skin or around your abdomen. Fat has a soft appearance.

The human body is in its prime from puberty until your early thirties. Prime means your body can build and maintain muscle mass easily. Your body needs the most calories during these years and burns them up easily and efficiently. It is no surprise then that the majority of athletes and sportspersons are known to be at their best from teenage years until around the age of 30.

Building and maintaining muscle mass is a combination of **keeping active and hormones** (chemical messengers in the human body), testosterone in men and growth hormone in both men and women.

Growth hormone stimulates growth, cell production and regeneration. The rate of Growth Hormone secretion from the pituitary* gland is highest around puberty when growth is rapid. Levels of growth hormone slowly decline, as we get older. It is widely recognised that the human body gradually begins to age sometime after thirty years. The aging human body, particularly over sixty years, is defined by a slow loss of muscle mass, loss of bone density and an increase in the amount of stored fat (25).

Pituitary gland is located at the base of the skull underneath the brain, behind the bridge of the nose.

An excess of fat covers up muscle definition. Doing sit ups when you are overweight will improve muscle strength but won't give you a visible six pack.

Ultimately, a leaner body shape can only be achieved by losing excess fat and working your muscles with exercise or hard physical work.

Human bodies quickly and efficiently convert carbohydrate, protein and fat in food to energy it can use as fuel or as building blocks for new cells (metabolic rate). The metabolic rate gradually declines, as we get older. It slows at about 10% every ten years after the age of thirty. This means that a sixty-year-old needs about 25% less calories to maintain their body weight than they did when they were in their twenties.

Summary – Body Shape

- The shape you are as an adult is defined by the bone structure and muscle mass you inherited.
- Focusing on taking care of your body will help you accept the bits you cannot change and improve your body shape (build muscle, lose excess fat).

Part 2
When

Chapter 8
History

Why do we want to eat a lot?
Why do we become fat?

Humans have evolved over an estimated six million years.
During this time, humans have endured, by having children and teaching those children how to survive. **All life depends on access to nutrition and water. Our desire to eat and drink is programmed into our bodies (DNA) as 'survival'.** This ancient drive, to eat food when it's available is not going to go away. Nevertheless, you can be in charge of your primal urges and control the desire to eat.

For millions of years, the greatest amount of energy and physical strength humans needed was to search for, hunt and prepare food to eat.

Farming began around 10,000 BC from then on humans lived in an area rather than travelling over long distances to hunt and gather food. Humans stayed in one area to concentrate on growing crops and domesticating animals to eat. Farming involved hard physical labour and food production was dependent on the weather (19). People were most likely to die from infections or disease or starvation. Plus, if you were malnourished due to lack of food after a bad harvest, people would have been more likely to die if they picked up an infection or developed a disease.

Human survival depended on dedicating time to search for, prepare and eat food.

Subsequently, the brain and body evolved **continual stimulation** to eat when food is available. We have a natural drive to binge eat to get as much energy as we can when there is food around. After thousands of years of evolution, it's programmed into our brains to overeat. This makes it difficult to choose wisely and eat lower calorie foods. It also means when we are hungry, our brain keeps thinking about food and won't stop until we eat.

Why when people lose weight are they more likely to go back to old eating habits. Ending up re-gaining the weight they lost?

For thousands of years, the amount of food people could eat was ruled by the seasons and the weather.

Humans evolved to overeat during the warm and wet seasons, when more food was available. They would then store food left over from the harvests to eat during times when less food could be produced. If the weather had been bad, crops could be ruined and people would have to continue with the hard-physical labour of everyday life with very little food.

Wealthy countries have only had a wide variety of foods available all year round for about one hundred years. The human body and its **program of 'survival', which is see food, eat food, has not changed.**

This is important because we see this 'survival' pattern reflected in the way people 'diet'.

When people want to lose weight, the amount of food they eat is restricted and exercise is increased. Motivated people generally do well, feel good and have energy. They will be losing weight rapidly and feeling pleased with themselves.

Typically, eating less and being more active will last about three or four months and then people find their energy level starts to drop, feeling more tired and less motivated. People may not be aware of feeling hungry but start to find it harder to stop eating when they have a meal or snack.

We have evolved to function well through periods of less food and increased activity.

However, the human body only copes with this for a limited time, about three to four months. Then it relies on having access to more food to recover lost body weight. Humans have a long history of surviving through short periods of restrictive eating when less food is available.

Geography, seasonality, weather, climate, wars, civil unrest, poverty and disease influence the availability of food and water. Where and when food is grown, reared or caught has an impact on its accessibility. Seasons primarily dictate the food being grown or caught. Countries near to the equator have very mild seasons so would be more effected by climates, droughts, natural disasters, wars and poverty, than winter. The UK, Northern Europe and North America would have a history of less food availability during the winter months.

After about four months of losing weight, the 'dieter' is fighting against a body that adapts by slowing the rate it burns calories (metabolic rate). If a person is determined and sticks to their diet, the body responds to a prolonged state of famine* by further reducing the calories it uses to conserve. This makes a person feel more tired with a stronger drive to eat, so they start breaking their diet. The body is programmed 'to survive'; it wants to recover the weight it lost (26).

Slowing of the metabolic rate
Lowers energy levels and makes people feel grumpy, less tolerant and preoccupied with thoughts about food.

The body wants you to rest more to conserve energy so the food you eat can be stored rather than used up. It is very hard to remain motivated to continue 'dieting' at this point. Even the most disciplined of us will plan to stick to the diet but it would take only one overeating episode to 'blow it' like having a meal out or planning to eat one biscuit then eating ten. Once episodes of breaking the diet start to happen, your brain will drive you to repeat old eating habits to restore the weight you lost.

Dieting does not work long term because we are expecting our body to cope with the demands of everyday life, plus exercise, whilst restricting the energy it gets from food.

Famine – not enough food, scarcity, shortage

Summary – History

- Humans have survived and grown to be the dominant species on earth because they spend time and effort on producing and eating food.
- The human body copes with food restriction (dieting) with increased activity (exercise) for about four months. After this, it switches to survival mode, slowing the rate it uses up calories making you feel tired and hungry.
- Dieting does not maintain weight loss long term. Most people regain all the weight they lost and more within six months to one year after starting a diet.
- After four months or more of 'dieting', fatigue sets in.

Chapter 9
Why Does Fatigue Matter?

Fatigue is the feeling of being physically and mentally tired.

Everyone gets tired its natural.

Fatigue is different from feeling drowsy or apathetic

Fatigue is:

Reduced or no energy

Physical or mental exhaustion

Lack of motivation

Made worse by one or more of...

Strenuous exercise or a physically demanding job

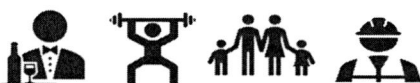

Emotional stress: anxiety, depression, caring for others, a mentally demanding job

Boredom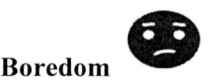

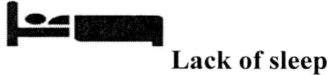**Lack of sleep**

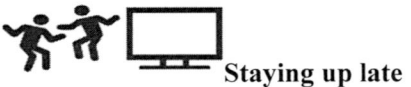 Staying up late

Having too much caffeine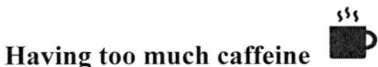

Drinking too much alcohol, makes you feel tired and hungry
Once effect of alcohol has worn off it has a depressive effect on mood

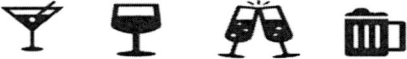

Eating lots of readymade, high calorie snacks and takeaway food especially late at night
Body has to deal with digesting food and storing energy when it should be resting

Eating less than your body needs to function well (dieting or disordered eating) and doing regular intense exercise

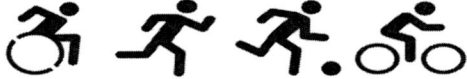

If your current lifestyle involves several of the behaviours listed above, you probably suffer with fatigue, felt most strongly in the evenings, especially at the end of the week.

Fatigue is a problem if you want to lose weight because it's difficult to feel motivated to change eating and activity behaviours if you feel physically and mentally drained. Plus, fatigue is more likely to keep someone trapped in a cycle of **trigger, behaviour, reward.**

So...

When humans restrict what they eat, there is rapid weight loss for a few weeks. Then the rate of weight loss slows as the body gradually lowers its metabolic rate to conserve loss of energy. Your body does this because it is responding to a state of prolonged starvation or 'famine'. It adapts to use less energy so that you can live long enough to get food. It does not matter how much body fat you have; the human body is programmed to conserve energy to survive.

Over thousands of years of history, the body has evolved to preserve fat to survive through famine, physical hardship or pregnancy.

When the human body is in a state of starvation (prolonged dieting), it will (26):

- **breakdown muscle as well as fat to use as energy**
- make you **tired so that you sit around more** and are not using up so many calories moving around
- **think about food** to drive you to search for and eat food as a priority over anything else. That is why when people feel hungry, the brain is preoccupied with strong reoccurring thoughts about food.

There is usually rapid weight loss in the early days of dieting as the body loses a combination of stored glucose from muscles and liver (glycogen), muscle tissue (protein) and some fat. So, **people who repeat cycles of 'yoyo' dieting will with each episode lose muscle mass and some fat. When they go back to old eating habits and regain weight, they will regain fat not recover muscle***. This leaves them with a body that no longer has as many calorie burning muscle cells as it did before they started dieting.

*rapid weight loss is associated with muscle wasting as well as loss of fat. Muscle will recover but it takes longer and relies on the person keeping active.

If you want to lose body fat:

- **Do not go on a diet**
- **Change your eating habits**

Chapter 10
How to Control Your Desire for Food (Appetite)

Hunger is the physical need for energy (food)

After we wake up, our body needs extra energy for movement and our brain uses more energy to be alert and have clear thoughts. A combination of the brain and hormones (*chemical messengers*) stimulate the desire to eat every 4 to 6 hours when we are awake. This is the **hunger cycle**.

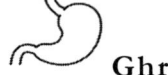Ghrelin

The main hunger-stimulating hormone. It is secreted from the **stomach** and circulates to your brain where it **triggers the drive to eat**. When the stomach is empty and blood sugar is low, and when people haven't eaten in several hours, the stomach produces more **ghrelin**, this makes us feel hungry.

Leptin

After eating, a hormone called **Leptin** which is made by **fat cells**, works to **reduce appetite**, this stops us wanting to eat.

If the body is sleep deprived (inconsistent and poor quality), the level of **ghrelin** rises rapidly, and fat cells produce less **leptin**. This makes you feel hungry and drives you to eat (27).

These body processes are complicated involving a lot of glands and hormones. It's helpful to have some knowledge of what happens in your body, but you didn't buy this book to study physiology so I will just write about the important hormones.

The most important hormone that makes your body store energy is insulin.

Insulin is a hormone.

Made by the pancreas. Special cells called the **Islets of Langerhans produce insulin**. After you eat any food that contains carbohydrate, once digested, it **enters the bloodstream* as glucose**.

*Blood is the transport system for your body driving around the oxygen and nutrients your body needs to live.

Insulin's job is like a key

It opens up your body cells to let glucose in which is then used for energy. Glucose is very important to your body as the main *fast fuel* for muscles (movement) and your brain (thinking).

There is always a little bit of insulin floating around in our bloodstream 24 hours a day. This stops your blood glucose level getting too high and keeps it at a level the body functions best (3.5-6 mmol/L). Plus, your body can take in glucose for energy whenever it needs it.

This bit is important

When people digest carbohydrate foods, there is a surge in the blood glucose level. The pancreas releases extra insulin to quickly move the glucose from blood into body cells.

When there are higher levels of insulin in the blood, the body switches to 'energy storage mode' and stops releasing stored glucose and fat.

'Energy storage'

After we eat, the body keeps some of the energy (calories) for later by topping up glucose and fat stores. This stored glucose and fat should then be released in-between meals and overnight when you are not eating. This ensures the body has access to energy for body function day and night.

Insulin moves glucose from the blood into body cells.

It does this without any problems if you are a healthy weight and keep active. On the other hand, if your lifestyle means that you sit around most of the day and have become overweight, insulin doesn't work as well. This is **insulin**

resistance. As you gain more **abdominal** (belly) **fat,** the body **resists insulin** and it's harder for insulin to open up body cells to let glucose enter. **It's like the key no longer fits the lock.**

When **insulin** cannot do its job properly, the blood glucose remains higher for longer after you eat. Your pancreas will keep responding to higher blood glucose levels by releasing more and more insulin until blood glucose goes down to normal.

Your body functions best if it can keep the blood glucose level between 3.5– 6 mmol/L. If a person has insulin resistance, it's harder for the body to clear glucose from the blood. Over time, people with worsening insulin resistance can develop **glucose intolerance** and then **type 2 diabetes.**

The **problem with high levels of insulin in the blood for longer after eating is it keeps the body in a state of 'energy storage'.**

High levels of insulin **'signal' the body to stop releasing glucose and fat and to store the energy from any food eaten.**

The **consequence** of this is that **one or two hours after eating a person feels tired and hungry again so eats food** they do not need. This is because their body has not switched back to energy release and is stuck in storage mode. This creates a **vicious cycle of hunger, lack of energy, weight gain. People may feel a sense of despair that they cannot lose weight** (28)

Vicious Cycle

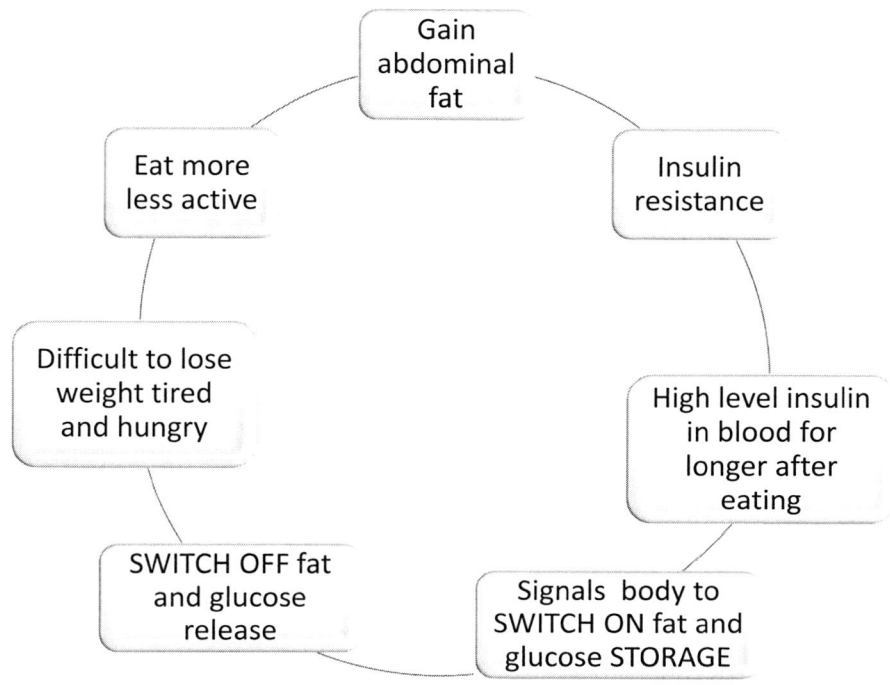

People want to eat all the time and feel tired
because they are overweight

The way to **break this cycle** is to eat in a way that holds a **stable blood glucose level.**

- Achieved by eating **controlled portions** of **low GI carbohydrates**
- Planning **balanced meals** and becoming **more active**

Exercise speeds up the release of stored energy (glucose and fat)
Exercise makes body cells more receptive to insulin
Exercise reduces insulin resistance

What causes weight gain and prevents loss of fat?

Regularly eating more calories than your body needs to function

Moving too little
An inactive lifestyle

Responding to hunger rather than trying to control it
Eating what you want when you want

If you have strong emotional triggers to eating
- *Anxiety and depression*
- *Binge eating disorder*
- *Comfort eating*

Do you need psychological support/treatment?

All or nothing thinking
If you eat too much one day – think 'I've blown it'.
Make excuses for yourself to relapse back into old behaviours

Not taking full responsibility for what you eat
Making excuses, blaming family, friends, co-workers, food manufacturers, restaurants, takeaways for giving you too much food.

Most of your social and or work life centres around eating or drinking alcohol

If you have a habit of drinking alcohol most evenings – more than 1 large glass wine 250ml or a pint of beer/lager/ale or double measure of spirit 50ml

How to lower insulin resistance to lose fat

Start being more active
Introduce some regular exercise that you like

Controlled portions of low GI carbohydrate in meals (see what section)

Choose to eat more foods that are known to be beneficial to your health

Don't add extra sugar to drinks or food
No sweets made mainly from sugar
No drinks especially fizzy drinks that contain sugar – includes concentrated fruit juice

Balanced meals and snacks.
Slows speed that glucose enters your blood stream. Need less insulin to deal with it

Plan and stick to structured meals and snacks

Don't eat or drink anything that contains calories for 12 to 14 hours overnight
Best time to fast 19.00 to 07.00

Want to lose weight quickly? Yoyo dieter? 18-hour fast. Eat two balanced meals within a 6-hour period, no snacks or desserts. Stick to weight loss calories. When you have had enough of 18-hour fasting, go back to 12 hours fasting from 7 pm until 7 am, with weight maintenance calories. This will maintain muscle mass, losing body fat on the 18-hour fasting days.

Disordered Eating pattern

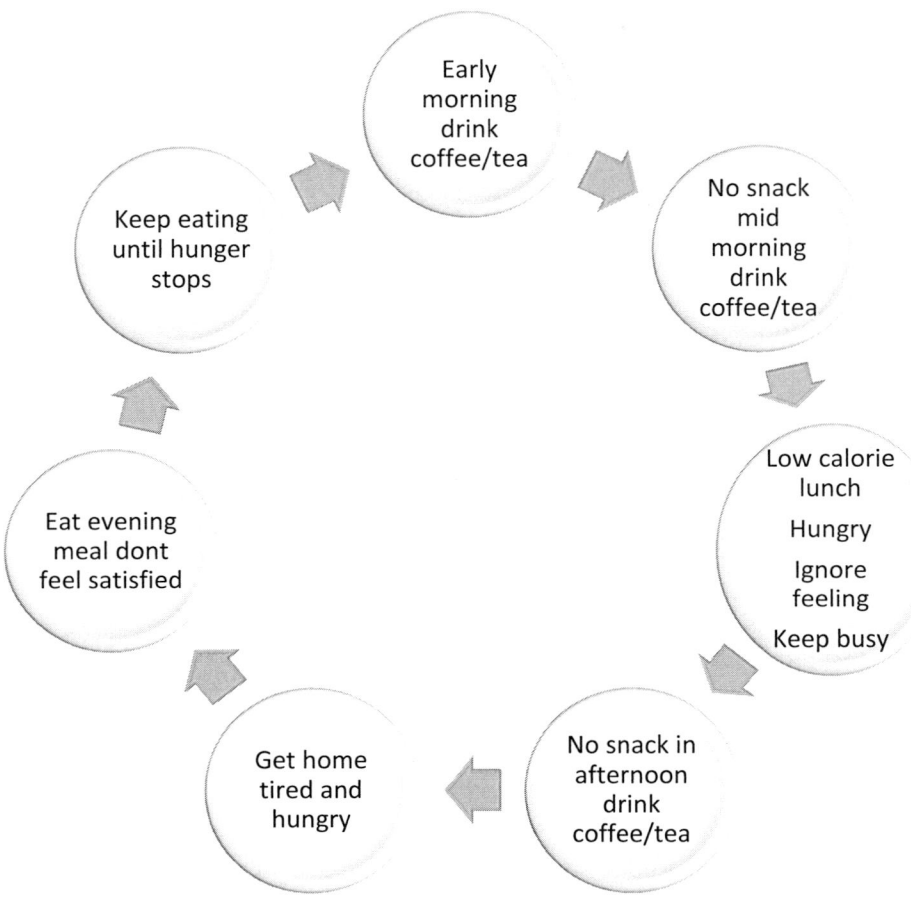

- o **This eating pattern is disordered because it has no structure**
  The pattern is restriction with a period of excessive eating. After virtually no food for most of the daytime, their brain will be totally focused on driving them to eat.
- o **Restrictive eating triggers cravings for food**

Typically, any time around mid-afternoon to early evening.

The brain drives you to eat because its energy stores of glucose (stored as glycogen) have dropped low over the course of the day. This person will eat and keep eating until all the food is digested. It takes up to two hours to fully digest a meal. People can consume a lot of calories in two hours. Craving for food won't stop until their brain registers that energy stores are topped up and switches off the drive to eat.

When 'cravings' happen

It's natural to desire foods that are high in fat and sugar because they are energy dense (contain lots of calories).

The trouble with this?

Less likely to select heathier choices that take longer to prepare. More likely to eat ready-made foods at a **fast pace**. People may end up eating more calories over a couple of hours than if they ate three balanced meals throughout the day.

It's easy to get into this pattern with busy work and family lives. Plus, cramming in all your calories in the evening over two to four hours stops you feeling hungry the next morning, so continues the same pattern of disordered eating.

If this disordered pattern of eating continues, it could lead to **binge eating** where the person has a **sense of no control over the amount they eat**. Even though eating is a great pleasure, binges leave people feeling guilty because of the loss of control and fear of weight gain. This is more likely to keep you in the **cycle of restrictive dieting in the daytime with overeating in the evening**.

The evening is the worst time to consume a lot of food because people are tired at the end of the day and more likely to sit on the sofa for several hours and then go to bed.

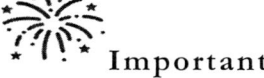 Important

While we sleep, the human body deals with **repairing damaged cells, getting rid of waste products and building new cells because it does not have to prioritise thinking and movement.**

The body's natural restoration processes will be limited if it is dealing with digesting and storing of food late evening or during the night.

Try to get a routine of eating and do not eat too late too often. Ideally, no food after seven in the evening; *see fasting*.

If a person eats when they feel like it with no structure, their brain is more likely to move from **hunger to appetite to cravings**

HUNGER	APPETITE	CRAVINGS
Physical need for energy every four to six hours when humans are awake	Long periods between meals without food	Inadequate food eaten during daytime
Natural hunger cycle	Brain starts becoming preoccupied with thoughts of food	Strong thoughts about food
	Feel tired	Eats late afternoon or early evening more likely to overeat and keep eating until feels satisfied
	Hunger pangs	
	Desire food	Brain drives people to eat foods high in fat and sugar

When you are craving food, it's very difficult to stop yourself from overeating.

Example of a Structured eating pattern

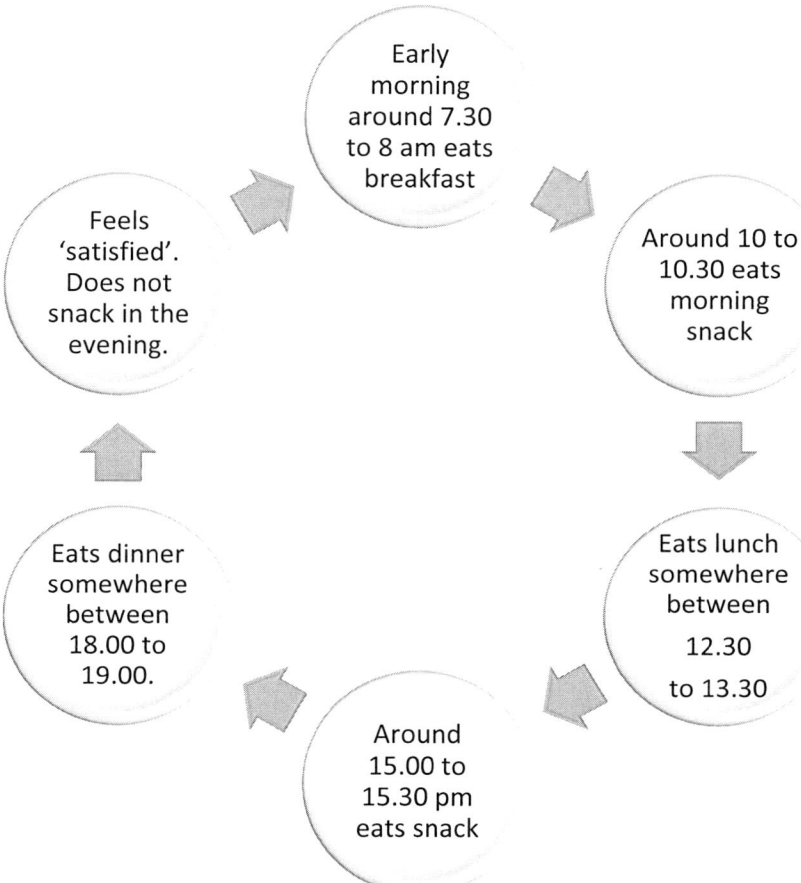

A simple routine of eating will give this person's body the energy and nutrients (protein, vitamins and minerals) that it needs to function well. Because this person has eaten at regular intervals around the 4- to 6-hour physical need for energy cycle, they have satisfied hunger and are in control of their appetite. This person is more likely to maintain a stable weight, lose body fat and gain muscle if they are more active.

If you travel to any country in the world, the majority of the population will have an eating pattern of two or three meals a day. If they eat only one or two small meals, this is unlikely to be by choice, rather the result of poverty.

Two to three meals a day with one to two snacks in-between meals gives people the energy they need to move around, think clearly and get work done.

Reminder – the human body has evolved to tolerate restrictive eating for short periods, about three to four months after that fatigue sets in.

Think about your routine of eating. Write down what you eat and when for a few days, this will show you the reality of your eating pattern.

Summary – How to control your appetite

It can become a battle of will power to keep dieting

- ❖ Eating regular meals make fat cells release **Leptin,** which **reduces your appetite,** so you eat less.
- ❖ Eating regular meals at similar times reduces the amount of **Ghrelin** secreted from the stomach, so people **feel less hungry, eating less food.**
- ❖ Getting **consistent quality sleep** stops the level of **Ghrelin** rising. This stops a person feeling so hungry.
- ❖ **Controlled portions of low GI carbohydrate** foods keep the **level of insulin** low in blood. This means the body can **switch quickly** from **storing** glucose and fat after a meal to **releasing** it

If you feed your body properly, it will settle into a pattern of eating and regulate the amount you eat. You won't need to diet any more.

Chapter 11
Fasting

Humans have fasted throughout history

Mainly for religious festivals or as part of spiritual discipline or cleansing. In addition, it is common knowledge that when people suffer from illness or disease, they may lose their appetite, eating less while they are unwell.

Human beings have thousands of years of experience with periods of no food or very little food

Typically, famine caused by poor harvests, wars or poverty. Humans have developed bodies that cope well with short periods of little or no food. Humans have not evolved to cope with food restriction or dieting over a long time.

Not everyone can tolerate no food for a whole day, let alone several days. So, there are different types of fasting to suit most people.

Fasting is beneficial

Fasting **switches the body to use mainly stored body fat.** This happens when stores of glycogen (glucose) are depleted.

Fasting is reported to improve blood glucose control, help suppress your appetite and maintain muscle mass by abstaining from eating or drinking any calories (food energy) overnight from between 12 to 18 hours (55).

What happens to our bodies while we fast?

The majority of functions in the human body are to maintain good health and ensure our survival. Humans have evolved with the experience of living through famine. Our bodies know that periods with no food result in muscle loss. Muscle loss makes us weaker and less able to move around, find and prepare food. So, the body releases more **growth hormone**, this maintains a hormone called insulin like growth factor (IGF-1). IGF-1 promotes growth of body cells, especially skeletal muscle.

This means, fasting protects muscle mass and switches your body to using body fat as its main source of energy.

Want to lose fat fast?

Try **fasting for 18 hours**. This means no food, only water or drinks that are calorie free. Eating two meals within a six-hour period during the daytime; no snacks, no desserts.

Evidence is accumulating that eating in a six-hour period and fasting for eighteen hours can trigger a **metabolic switch** from **glucose-based** (carbohydrates and protein) to **ketone-based** (fat) energy; with decreased inflammation, increased longevity and decreased incidence of diseases including cancer (53).

18-hours too long?

If eighteen-hour fasting does not work for you or you gave it ago but ended up eating. Then **12-hour overnight fasting** is beneficial and achievable.

- 12-hour overnight fasting helps to control your appetite during the daytime, maintains muscle mass, and helps keep off any lost body fat.
- The optimum time for overnight fasting is **seven in the evening to seven in the morning**. See if you can manage **14 hours** on some days in the week.
- This is not always possible if you work late or eat out in the evening, so if dinner is later, you should still do the full **12 hours fasting**, for example, finish eating around 9 pm, do not eat anything until after 9 am the next day.
- Digesting food is demanding on our bodies. After we eat, the priority is to use the energy from the food for body functions for two hours and any excess food energy is stored for later.

Reminder – the more we spread eating out over the day, the longer our bodies need to switch on energy storage and switch off energy release. Bodies need at least 12 hours overnight with no food to switch to releasing stored body fat for energy (54).

During sleep, our body regenerates by building new cells, getting rid of old or dead cells and waste products. It manages this efficiently if it's not having to deal with digesting and storing energy from food.

When the body uses fat for energy

The breakdown of body fat releases **ketone bodies. Ketone bodies** have an effect of **suppressing your appetite**. Once the body is using more stored body fat for energy, hunger will feel weaker around mealtimes, with a quicker sense of satisfaction after eating lighter meals or snacks. This keeps the body in a natural four to six-hour hunger cycle with **internal triggers**, signalling the physical need for energy. When the body is releasing stored fat, it suppresses appetite and, more importantly, stops us from craving foods high in fat and sugar.

Overnight 12-hour fasting is hard for the first two to three weeks; you will go to bed feeling hungry. **Be determined**, your body will get used to not eating after 7 pm and your brain will stop thinking about food in the evening.

Fasting means no food or drinks that contain calories, so that includes alcohol and milk in tea or coffee.

❖ **Fasting is beneficial for twelve hours overnight every day**.

If you are successful in sticking to this, you will lose up to ½ a stone or 7 lbs of fat in the first few weeks. This helps lower insulin resistance and helps suppress appetite in the daytime.

Reminder – If you **want to lose body fat quickly,** say for a special event and feel you can be disciplined, then **increase the fasting period up to 18-hours**.

- This means **no food at all, or drinks that contain calories for 18 hours once a day**
- Then eat two balanced meals within a six-hour period (see balanced meal section): no snacks, no desserts
- Do this for as long as you can tolerate it
- Then go back to overnight fasting for 12 hours from 7 pm to 7 am, with three balanced meals or two balanced meals, with one or two snacks between meals.

If you have a history of binge eating, I would advise you to focus on the twelve hours overnight fasting with ordered balanced meals during the daytime. Longer periods without food are likely to trigger binge episodes and may put you back into a pattern of disordered restriction then bingeing.

*This book **does not** promote total fasting for short periods of up to five days. This means no calories from food or drinks 24-hours a day. It's difficult to do and should be under the guidance and monitoring of a doctor or dietitian.*

People who are underweight (BMI less than 18.5) or women who are pregnant should not fast longer than 12 hours overnight.

Summary – Fasting

- ❖ Overnight fasting works by making your body switch to using mainly body fat for energy. People lose up to ½ stone or 7 lb or 3–4 kg over a few weeks with consistent adherence to 12-hour fasting. Any loss of body fat achieved through healthy eating habits and exercise will stay off, if overnight fasting is maintained.

- ❖ When a body uses more stored body fat for energy, it helps suppress your appetite during the daytime, so people cope better with eating smaller structured meals and snacks.

- ❖ If you want to lose weight quickly for a special event, increase the overnight fasting to 18-hours a day. Eating two balanced meal within a 6-hour period, no snacks, no desserts. Aim for a weight loss calorie intake (see chapter on energy).

Chapter 12
Ordered Eating

Ordered eating is normal eating.

So, what's normal?

Definition of normal is *'in a typical or structured way' (1)*.

Reminder – the natural hunger cycle is every four to six hours once we are awake. If we give our body what it needs to function well, it will regulate consumption for us. We won't feel deprived of food or yoyo from restriction to overeating.

Write down examples of what you eat and when on a typical day; one weekday and one day over the weekend. This helps to focus on the reality of your eating pattern.

Do you have ordered or disordered eating?

If your life is busy or chaotic, with food fitted in around the demands of work or family. It would be wise to plan realistic time windows when you are most likely to be able to eat.

If you are thinking 'I can't do that' then you may not be ready to change eating habits.

Remember that your lifestyle and eating habits are keeping you overweight
Change is difficult but not impossible

Speak to the people closest to you and ask if they are willing to make some healthy changes to the way they eat so you can support each other.

Example of disordered eating:

- A person gets up early before work has thirty minutes to get ready, doesn't feel hungry, doesn't eat breakfast, drinks a coffee.
- Arrives at work has another coffee.
- Works through to lunchtime. Sometimes gets a sandwich or salad to eat at desk, sometimes keeps working and doesn't eat.
- Drinks coffee and tea through the day, has a couple of biscuits.
- Early evening, gets home. Aware of stronger feelings of hunger, feels tired and grumpy. Low motivation to cook so snacks and heats up a ready meal. Thinks 'I haven't eaten much today so I can eat what I want'.
- Spends much of the evening in front of the TV because they feel tired, starts snacking. Opens share bag of crisps, intends to have a few but finishes whole packet. Drinks two large glasses of wine to unwind.
- Gets up next day and repeats the same pattern.

This person has got into a pattern that prioritises work, they are not caring well for their body.

A full life is a combination of work, socialising, entertainment and relaxation.

If this person gave their body the nutrition it needs to function well, they would have more energy particularly in the evening to be involved in other interests and activities. **Personal interests outside of work or family enhance our lives, making it more enjoyable and worthwhile.**

Be aware of fatigue, once that creeps in motivation for life drops.

People with disordered patterns of eating may feel like they never have enough time to do the things they want to or the energy to exercise or play sports. This can leave people resenting the demands of their job or family, imagining how much better life would be if they did not have to work or care for others.

Humans are resilient and great problem solvers

- ❖ **The majority of people can deal with the complicated demands of life**
- ❖ **Prioritise caring for yourself and everything else will get easier because you will feel healthier and in control of your body**

❖ Another way of putting it is, care for yourself as much as you would care for someone else or your work

Why do I need a time window to eat?

Time windows bring order into your eating routine.

Write down your typical daily routine. Breakfast is important because it is like putting wood on the fire of the body's metabolism. Basically, if you eat breakfast, you will have more energy, burn calories more efficiently during the day and have more control over your appetite, particularly late afternoon.

Planning when and what to eat in advance focuses attention on the best times to nourish your body. If people write down a simple plan, they are more likely to stick to it.

Not everyone suits eating first thing in the morning. *Write down time windows when you know you will be able to eat; 30 minutes for a snack and one hour for a meal.* This is flexible enough to allow a routine that is ordered but not ridged. As long as you have food and have started to eat during the window, you will be keeping to the plan.

Remember the four to six-hour hunger cycle. Don't leave eating the next meal longer than six hours. **Be aware of times of the day you feel hunger more strongly.** If you find you are still feeling driven to snack in the evening, add a snack in mid-afternoon, this will take the edge off your hunger in the evening and control your appetite.

It only works if you stick to your plan. Sometimes you will need to eat even if you do not feel hungry.

Summary – Ordered Eating

❖ Write down a typical day, what you eat and when. It helps to pay attention to your pattern of eating and start planning 'time windows'; thirty minutes for a snack and one hour for a meal.

❖ Flexible time windows are important to bring order into your eating pattern. Aim for two to three balanced meals, with one to two snacks a day, between meals.

❖ It is very important to stick to time windows and eat meals and snacks when you planned. Sometimes you must eat even if you do not feel hungry, especially in the morning.

Part 3
What

Chapter 13
Foods You Can Swap for a Healthier Alternative

No one is perfect. When foods are banned or considered 'bad' or only for treats, we deprive ourselves of meals, snacks and desserts we enjoy. Rather than banning foods, consider swapping to an equally tasty healthy alternative.

Foods that need swapping for healthier alternatives	Why and What
AVOID **Sugary drinks especially fizzy drinks.** **Adding extra sugar into drinks or on food.** **Foods that are mainly made from sugar, sweets.** **Foods that have sugar as the first or second listed ingredient. Includes some breakfast cereals.**	**Why?** These are **fast carbohydrates** – Raise your blood glucose level rapidly, needs a lot of insulin to deal with it. <u>Instead</u> Tea or coffee with no added sugar, water, herbal teas and slice of orange, lemon or lime to a glass of water. Drink milk or have a cappuccino or a latte as a snack. **Small amounts of high sugar foods** added onto other sugar free foods are okay, such as teaspoon of jam or honey on natural yogurt or porridge. Small bar or a few squares of a good quality chocolate
AVOID	**Why?**

Fructose – a sugar in fruit juice, honey and processed foods that contain derivatives of maize or corn Look at the label of the foods you eat regularly if glucose-fructose-corn syrup is in the ingredients, start looking for an alternative.

Our bodies deal with glucose, no problem. However, we have not evolved to deal with **large amounts** of **fructose.** When **fructose** gets to our liver, it is **converted into fat** (triglycerides). If the liver has to deal with a lot of fructose, it gets deposited as fat around your abdomen (visceral).

Instead

Have **whole fruits**. Smoothie rather than juice, because it's a mix of juice and whole fruit blended together
(200–300 ml/small or medium)

AVOID
High GI (glycaemic index) carbohydrate foods (see section on GI) Includes some ready-made gluten free foods. Gluten free is wheat, rye, barley or oats that have had the protein removed. All that is left is highly refined 'fast' carbohydrate; High GI.

Why?
Usually, **foods made from white flour (wheat or maize/corn) or a lot of sugar**. Highly processed (ground down then cooked) so easy to digest; causes rapid spike in your blood glucose level. Need a lot of insulin to deal with it.

Instead

Smaller **controlled portions of low GI starchy carbohydrate** foods (see GI section)

AVOID
Cheap solid fats – trans or hydrogenated fat or ghee (concentrated butter). Check labels on pastries, pies, cookies, cakes, pasties.

Why?
Liquid fats are turned into solid fats, creates an **un-naturally saturated fat**.
Some ready-made foods are made using **hydrogenated fat** because it takes longer to go off, so food has a longer sell by date

Instead

Whenever possible stick to eating fat that remains in its **natural state**
Liquid fats, the best is cold pressed or extra virgin olive and vegetable oils or nut and seed oils. This includes **natural solid fats** (saturated) like butter, cream, coconut, fat in

meat, poultry, egg yolks. The **human body has had thousands of years eating and digesting these fats without a problem**.

Rather than frying food, add fat after.

Boiled potatoes with butter, or drizzle on oil.

Potato wedges or chips dry roasted then toss in olive oil.

Fat in a meal helps you to feel satisfied or 'full' for longer after eating.

For snacks or desserts, add cream or full fat natural yogurt or nuts or some quality chocolate (high % cocoa solids)

Why?

AVOID
Sweeteners
Artificial chemicals
Includes Agave nectar, plus it's high in fructose.

Not digestible – The body cannot digest sweeteners, so cannot use them for energy.

The bacteria inside the bowel feed off sweeteners. This generates gas, causing bloating and flatulence. Too much gas fills the bowel and stretches it; can cause sharp 'colicky' pain.

If consumed in excessive amounts, sweeteners have a laxative effect.

Using sweeteners **keeps you addicted** to intensely sweet foods. You can adapt taste buds to prefer foods and drinks without added sugar.

No added sweeteners. **No diet fizzy drinks**.

<u>**Instead**</u>

Foods that contain natural sugar, fresh fruit or dried fruit.

Be determined to fight the urge for sweet tastes. Your taste buds will, after about two weeks, get used to the real taste of food and drink without artificial sweeteners.

If you stop adding sweeteners but still drink diet fizzy drinks, you will keep yourself attached to craving intensely sweet food and drinks

AVOID

Cheap sweets and chocolate
Sweets that contain mainly
sugar; toffee, fudge, boiled
sweets, children's sweets.
Chocolate that contains
sugary fillings

Why?

These are mainly made from sugar. **Don't buy chocolate if sugar is the first ingredient listed.**

<u>Instead</u>

'Quality not quantity'

Buy **high quality** chocolate. Good quality chocolate is nutritious (contains nutrients that are beneficial to your health)

❖ Chocolate covered nuts are a healthier and lower GI alternative.

❖ Watch the calories.

❖ Chocolate and nuts are energy dense. You need to know your calorie ranges and stick to it.

AVOID

Processed meat.
Any meat that has been
preserved by curing, salting,
smoking, drying or canning
or adding chemical
preservatives; sausages, hot
dogs, salami, ham, cured
bacon, corned beef, beef
jerky.
No leftover bits of carcass
meat (mechanically
recovered meat) ground up
and formed into processed
shaped meat, like sausages
or meat slices for
sandwiches, cheap pies or
meat pasties.
Fried, grilled or barbecued.
Any meat that has been
cooked or burnt at very
high temperatures.

Why?

Linked with higher risk of developing colon cancer, type-2 diabetes and heart disease.

Cooking at very high temperatures forms chemicals in the food that are damaging to our bodies.

<u>Instead</u>

'Quality not quantity'

Buy less cheap meat, chicken or fish

Buy joints of meat, chicken or fish on the bone. Cuts, fillets, a steak, sliced meat from a joint or offal that has been cut from an animal, chicken or fish.

Buy a whole fish or chicken.

Include more vegetarian meals using peas, beans or lentils as the protein portion in your meal.

*If having **'meaning and purpose'** helps you to change your eating habits, buy organic and free range. Try being a flexitarian or vegetarian or choose more plant-based meals,* *especially if you want to reduce your carbon footprint and are against cruelty to animals.*

Summary – Foods you can swap for a healthier alternative

❖ Cut out sugary drinks and foods that are made mainly from sugar. Allow your taste buds to get used to food and drinks without added sugar or sweeteners

❖ No concentrated fruit juices. Daily limit of one glass, 200ml, fresh juice or smoothies

❖ No foods with added glucose fructose corn syrup; check listed ingredients on packaging

❖ Swap the starchy carbohydrates you eat the most often (rice, bread, potatoes) for a low GI alternative

❖ Choose to eat fats in their most natural state; not cooked at high temperatures or processed

❖ Buy the best quality food products you can afford

❖ Give up eating sweets and chocolate that are made mainly from sugar (1st ingredient listed).

If you struggle to give up intensely sweet foods, **fast for 18-hours for one day. Eat two balanced meals within a 6-hour period; no food or drinks that contain sugar for 24 hours**.

This works to reset your taste buds.

After a fast, taste buds will become more **sensitive to subtle flavours** so you can start to **enjoy healthy foods again**.

Chapter 14
Which Foods are Healthy and Why?

Choosing to eat healthier foods is a **powerful positive action** to being in control of your own health.

If we eat more nutrient-rich foods, we give our bodies what they need to function well.

Nutrients are parts of food that human bodies need to maintain and build new cells. There are **two types of nutrients, macro and micro**. Macro means large, micro means small.

The **Macronutrients are carbohydrates, fats and protein.**

Micronutrients are vitamins and minerals.

All living organisms need energy for movement and growth. Carbohydrate, fat and protein are the energy used to drive body function and thinking. Macronutrients are also part of the building blocks for cells in the body. Protein is important as part of the structure. Fat is part of the membranes (covering or sheath) of cells and works to keep body fluid in the right places.

Vitamins and minerals cannot be used for energy but are needed to convert the energy from carbohydrates, fats and proteins to a fuel our body can use. Vitamins and minerals are part of the structure of the human body, a good example is calcium in our bones and teeth.

The best vitamins and minerals are natural, contained inside food rather than in vitamin tablets. Vitamins are absorbed easily from your gut if they are a part of food. Vitamin and mineral tablets that are taken without food do not get absorbed and eventually exit your bowel.

In every meal or snack, aim to have at least two foods rich in nutrients that are beneficial for your health.

Beans, peas and lentils source of protein for vegetarians and vegans

Add substance and texture to a meal. High in fibre, 'filling'

Any Fish

Excellent lean protein, healthy fat especially

omega-3 in oily fish

Meat on the bone, cuts, joints or fillets (not cheap processed meat)

Source of protein, iron and B vitamins; digests slowly, gives filling and satisfying feeling in stomach

Any nuts and seeds

Packed with vitamins, minerals and healthy fats.

(except for nut allergies) nuts are beneficial to health.

Cows milk, cheese and eggs

Dairy foods are high in protein, calcium, B vitamins and minerals. A glass of milk is low calorie low fat and nutrient dense

(low GI food)

The quality of protein in any food is compared to the protein in egg

All vegetables – it's common for some people to dislike the taste of vegetables. Children have immature taste buds so are less likely to enjoy vegetables

As Children grow into adults and experience different foods and flavours its normal to develop a taste for a wider variety of vegetables and fruit

If you are an adult 'fussy eater' stick with the vegetables and fruit you do like and include them in your meals

Vegetables can be hidden and enhance the flavour of a meal if its mixed in – stews, casseroles, sauces, pasta sauces

Roasting vegetables tends to sweeten them which makes the taste more appealing. Add gravy, sauce or season

Sometimes the texture of hard vegetables puts people off or they may find it difficult to chew or swallow hard food – vegetables soften if they are cooked in stews or casseroles or canned

All fruits – try to eat the whole fruit when possible.

Any of the fruit is better than no fruit so if you prefer it peeled or stewed or tinned or a smoothie it's still beneficial to your health.

Common foods that add flavour, believed to have health benefits

Garlic (31) – Known for centuries for disease fighting properties. Contains Allicin reported to lower blood pressure and LDL cholesterol (LDL is risk factor for heart disease)

Seaweed – Low calorie, salty, crunchy. Source of protein, fibre and many vitamins and minerals. Small amount of fat is omega 3.

Ginger – long history of traditional/alternative medicine. Used to help digestion, reduce nausea, fight flu and colds

Blueberries – Low GI, adds flavour and colour. Low in calories. High in antioxidants, believed to help protect against aging and cancer.

Kale – mainly protein and fibre. Contains alot of vitamins, minerals and antioxidants *(stop free radicals that damage cells)* very low calorie content. Small amount of fat is omega 3

Turmeric – contains curcumin helps prevent heart disease, alzheimers and cancer (32, 33). Anti-inflammatory and antioxidant. Thought to improve symptoms of depression and arthritis

Summary – Which Foods are Healthy and Why?

- ❖ Choosing healthy foods is one of the most significant ways people can improve the health of their body.
- ❖ Include some vegetables, salad and fruit in every meal.
- ❖ Include nutrient dense foods in every meal; fish, meat, dairy foods, peas, beans or lentils, wholegrain rice or breads.

Chapter 15
Carbohydrate Foods and the GI

(Glycaemic Index)

Carbohydrates are important foods for energy

Glucose is the **'fast'** energy our bodies need for clear thought and for movement. Diets that cut out or restrict carbohydrates are extreme. Most people do not tolerate low carbohydrate diets for a long time.

Food is a great pleasure

Cutting out a whole food group, such as, carbohydrates is more likely to leave people feeling deprived. Denying yourself foods that you enjoy over a long time can result in episodes of overeating or binge eating (sense of losing control). Plus, it gets harder to avoid carbohydrates if you eat socially because you have limited choice or need a different meal to everyone else.

Living a long life

Research that looks at longevity, living a long life without developing a disease of aging (heart disease or cancer); report that populations whose diets are based on starchy carbohydrates, vegetables, fruit, peas, beans and lentils, live the longest (29). These diets (depending on the country) are a combination of wholegrain starchy carbohydrates, low GI green plantain, yams, beans, peas, lentils, vegetables, salad and fruit.

Digestion (34)

1. After we chew food and swallow, it enters the stomach which holds food. The stomach produces acid which kills off most of the bacteria, cleaning food.

2. The stomach then churns and squeezes food to break it down into a soup. This soup is released slowly in little spurts into your bowel, over one to two hours.

3. It is the small bowel's job to absorb the macronutrients and micronutrients from food. The liver makes enzymes which mix with the soup as it leaves the stomach and enters the bowel. Enzymes break up food into tiny pieces or into its building blocks, these can then be absorbed through the bowel wall.

4. The job of the small bowel is to absorb all the bits of food that can be used by the body.

5. Left over bits, water and fibre, enter your large bowel which absorbs water and salt to form compact stools. Stools get pushed to the bottom end of your bowel and are released down a toilet.

Low GI (35, 36)

If your meal is low GI, it takes longer for the gut to breakdown the food and absorb it into the bloodstream. This means the meal stays in the stomach for longer, making you feel full and satisfied, so it stops us eating too much.

Some low GI foods are more difficult for your digestive enzymes to break up. This means the carbohydrates are turned into glucose and absorbed slowly.

Glucose from low GI meals is absorbed slowly into the blood stream so it needs less insulin to deal with it. Lower levels of insulin in your blood mean more food is used up as energy and less is stored. Plus, there will be a **quicker switch from storing energy** after eating to **releasing** it.

Give your body regular energy with structured meals, eating at similar times. **Eat and repeat this pattern**. You will feel mild hunger before meals times and a sense of satisfaction from eating smaller portions of food.

A regular meal pattern keeps the 'flow' of short periods of energy storage, then a quick switch back to energy release. The body will settle into this rhythm of eating and not feel urges to overeat.

Remember this only works if you stick to a structured eating pattern

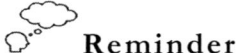

- ❖ The stomach and digestive enzymes made by the liver break food down to tiny pieces so that we can absorb it through the bowel wall.
- ❖ When carbohydrate foods such as wheat and corn are ground down to a fine flour or sugar is extracted from sugar cane, these will be digested very fast because the gut does not have much work to do.
- ❖ High GI foods are quick to digest so cause a rapid surge in your blood glucose level, matched with a rapid surge in insulin. **High insulin levels in the bloodstream switch off fat and glucose release and switch on storage of glucose and fat.**
- ❖ **High GI carbohydrates give a 'fast surge' of glucose energy which then drops as excess insulin moves it out of the blood into body cells. When a rapid surge in blood glucose drops back down, a person feels tired and hungry which drives them to eat again to get an energy lift.**

Sugar and high GI starchy carbohydrates are *fast carbohydrates*

***Fast carbohydrates* keep people in a cycle of feeling tired and hungry who gain weight easily and struggle to lose it**

Summary – Carbohydrate Foods and the GI (Glycaemic Index)

If you want to lose fat

- ❖ Cut out fast carbohydrates.
- ❖ Fast carbohydrates are any drinks that contain sugar, foods that contain mainly sugar where sugar is listed as the first ingredient, high GI starchy carbohydrates (foods made with white flour).
- ❖ Eat two or three regular meals every day.
- ❖ Eat at similar times every day. Once you are awake, do not leave it longer than six hours between meals.

❖ Control the portion of low GI carbohydrate. When you look at your meal, the amount of starchy carbohydrate should be no more than one third of what you are going to eat.

Chapter 16
Balanced Diet, Balanced Meals (37)

Why is having a balanced diet important?

- Balanced meals supply the nutrients your body needs to work effectively. Without balanced nutrition, human bodies are prone to infections, diseases and fatigue.
- Nutrition is essential for all body systems to function properly. Choosing healthy foods helps to maintain a healthy weight and reduce body fat. It gives people the energy for clear thinking and physical activity, to be able to do what they want. Balanced nutrition promotes better quality sleep and a sense of control over the health of your body.
- A balanced diet means eating a wide variety of foods in the right proportions. Gaining knowledge and practice in planning, preparing and serving the right amount of food is essential to achieve and maintain a healthy weight. Planning balanced meals is easier than you think and can quickly become a healthy habit.

What is a Balanced Meal?

When serving a meal onto a plate, it should be made up of roughly:

1/3 Starchy carbohydrate (low GI)
1/3 vegetables, salad or fruit
1/3 foods rich in protein

One or two portions of healthy fats – added or as part of food
Carbohydrates are any foods that contain starch or sugar

Starch is how plants store energy. The building blocks of starch is glucose. It does not taste sweet to us but when we digest it by breaking down food, it releases glucose.

Sugar is stored in plants as energy. The most farmed plants to produce sugar are sugar cane and sugar beet.

All carbohydrates give us sugar in the form of glucose. *We absolutely need glucose. Our brain and muscles function best with carbohydrates included in your diet.*

Slow carbohydrates (low GI) are the best choice.

Reminder – the amount of carbohydrate you need, especially fast carbohydrate (sugar or high GI starchy foods) depends on how active you are.

If your lifestyle is **inactive,** you do not need fast carbohydrates. Better to **swap for controlled amounts of starchy low GI carbohydrate**.

If you are obese (BMI greater than 30) and/or have type 2 diabetes or Polycystic ovary syndrome, **you should avoid** fast carbohydrates.

Swap Fast Carbs foods for Slow Carbs

Examples: **High GI** **'Fast carbohydrates'**	**Swap for low GI alternative** **'Slow carbohydrates'**	**Swap for lower calorie, low GI alternative**
Breakfast cereals Any processed (*ground down and formed into shapes*) Cornflakes Frosted flakes Coco pops	50g Muesli with fruit and/or nuts 50g Porridge 40g Multigrain flakes 50g Granola with fruit and/or nuts Shredded wheat X 2	30–50g portion of porridge oats served with fruit and milk or natural yogurt 2 egg omelettes

Examples: High GI 'Fast carbohydrates'	Swap for low GI alternative 'Slow carbohydrates'	Swap for lower calorie, low GI alternative
Rice Krispies Fruit and fibre Honey nut loops Crunchy clusters Puffed wheat Weetabix	40g Bran flakes with oat 40g Any high bran cereal – All bran *Dry weight*	1 slice granary bread with 2 eggs or lean bacon 2–3 slices 2 Rye crispbreads with low fat cream cheese or cottage cheese or 2 heaped teaspoons of a nut butter Sliced apple with 2 tsp nut butter
Rice	Basmati rice Wild rice Brown rice Risotto rice Bulgur wheat Couscous Quinoa *All 60g dry weight before cooking* *Or portion to 1/3 of meal plate*	Cauliflower rice Barley Mix rice with equal portion of any peas or beans; lowers GI and reduces calories in meal
Bread made from white flour **Any fish or meat in pastry or breadcrumbs or batter or covered in sugar-based sauce/marinade** **Pizza**	Wholegrain, granary bread seeded or nut (bread with bits in) **Fillings** – egg, tuna, salmon, chicken or meat (taken off a joint not processed sandwich meat), avocado and poached egg, cottage cheese with pineapple or apple slices Any wholemeal bread	Aubergine (eggplant) Thin seeded wholegrain or Oat cracker biscuits Choose small slices or small roll of Granary or Oatmeal bread with filling

Examples: High GI 'Fast carbohydrates'	Swap for low GI alternative 'Slow carbohydrates'	Swap for lower calorie, low GI alternative
	Pumpernickel bread Oatmeal/Oat bran bread Chapatti Sourdough bread Unprocessed Fish fillet or meat/poultry *(cut or joint or on bone)* Fajita – beef, chicken or vegetable Burrito – beef Corn Tortilla Small wholemeal pizza base *(size of side plate)* or toast oat or seeded wholegrain baguette, generous toppings	1 thick slice as an open sandwich or toast with topping
Mashed Potato **Jacket Potato** **Any potato that is ground up and formed into shapes** *Potato waffles, wedges, chips, bhajis, potato curry*	Boiled new potatoes or canned Roast, Jacket, microwaved *(limit to 2–3 egg sized potatoes or 1 mixed with root vegetables or 200–250g large potato)* Green plantain Elephant foot or purple or yellow yam Pakora – potato and cauliflower fried Cassava Sweet Potatoes – wedges, roasted or mash Jicama (Mexican turnip) Daikon radish Napa cabbage	Mashed turnip or swede Roasted root vegetables Carrots Parsnips Beetroot Onions Celery root Swede

Examples: **High GI** **'Fast carbohydrates'**	**Swap for low GI alternative** **'Slow carbohydrates'**	**Swap for lower** **calorie, low GI** **alternative**
Chips	Sweet potato wedges Baked lentil chips White or black bean chips Veggie chips	Kale chips
Crisps	30g Lentil crisps 30g Roasted chickpeas	30g Roasted peas 30g Salted popcorn
Currants, dates, figs **Lychees canned in** **syrup** **Cantaloupe melon,** **Galia melon** **Honeydew melon** **Watermelon**	Any other fruit	Any berries or a small apple
Broad beans **<u>Baked</u> sweet potato**	Any other vegetables, beans, peas or lentils Vegetable pate Vegetable bake Refried beans Lentil pie Lentil nut roast	**Any green** **vegetables** Cabbage Kale Spinach Watercress Spring greens Swiss chard Beet greens Bok choy Turnip greens Green beans Collard greens

Examples: High GI 'Fast carbohydrates'	Swap for low GI alternative 'Slow carbohydrates'	Swap for lower calorie, low GI alternative
		Green peppers Brussel sprouts Broccoli
Any white flour used for cooking/baking	Wholegrain or add seeds or nuts Mix half white flour with oats or almond or coconut flour Soya bean flour	Chickpea flour
Any Cannelloni Any lasagne Any quiche	Pasta of any shape White or wholemeal Spaghetti or macaroni Quinoa noodles Egg or rice noodles Vegetable moussaka Nut and vegetable roast	Zucchini stripes Kelp noodles (ground seaweed) 60g dry weight of soba noodles or fresh egg pasta filled with vegetables, meat or cheese
White Milk Dark Chocolate	High quality milk/white/dark chocolate	Mango Tinned peaches
Burger bun	Oatmeal or granary roll	Portobello mushroom
Sweets made mainly from sugar	Olives X 6 Nuts 20–30g Any fruit	Slices of apple Any berries Pineapple slices
Cake	Apple oat cake Banana bran muffins Small fruit muffin	2 or 3 mini bite size cakes squares; made with oats or high

Examples: High GI 'Fast carbohydrates'	Swap for low GI alternative 'Slow carbohydrates'	Swap for lower calorie, low GI alternative
		fruit, seed, nut and/or chocolate content
Majority of biscuits are high GI	Biscuits made from oats Chocolate coated oat biscuits Peanut/peanut butter cookies Biscuits made with a nut flour or with high nut content Cereal bars with fruit and/or nuts and chocolate	2 or 3 mini biscuit bites or 2 small biscuits; made with oats or high fruit, seed, nut and/or chocolate content
Majority of desserts are high GI **Keep portions small**	Individual fruit yogurt pot* Greek style yogurts fruit or honey* Fruit with yogurt or custard and sprinkle of nuts 15g, granola with ice cream or natural yogurt Small crepe with fruit and natural yogurt or custard	Natural yogurt Soya yogurt Coconut yogurt Custard with or without fruit Mousse – low fat Crème caramel *Small individual pots control calories or limit to 125g*

Yogurts without corners or layers of fruit jam, chocolate or biscuit pieces

Summary – Balanced diet, balanced meals

❖ The human body deals better with meals that digest slowly.

❖ Balanced meals give your body all the macro (energy and protein) and micronutrients (vitamins and minerals) it needs.

❖ When you eat a meal, all the foods are churned up together in the stomach. Protein, vegetables, salad or fruit, some fat, together with low

GI carbohydrate create a 'filling' meal that gives a slow release of energy and sense of satisfaction that controls appetite up until the next meal.

To lose excess belly fat, it helps if you know:

1. How to plan balanced meals that give your body what it needs to function well (energy, protein, vitamins and minerals). Meals that satisfy hunger and control appetite.
2. Roughly how many calories your body needs to maintain your current weight and have an idea of the number of calories in the foods you eat the most often (see section on energy).
3. How to ease into lifestyle changes overtime. Start with the changes to your eating habits that you believe will be the easiest to maintain (refer to sections on change and habits).

Chapter 17
Vegetables, Salad and Fruit

To date, all advice on healthy eating agrees that people should eat more vegetables, salad and fruit (30). These foods help our bodies function well, slow aging and have been shown to reduce the risk of developing cancer or heart disease or diabetes.

They are 'filling' and low calorie. Vegetables, salad and fruit provide carbohydrate but in small amounts that digest slowly. Plus, the vitamins and minerals contained in them are natural and absorbed into your body better than a vitamin tablet.

All vegetables, salad and fruit are good for you. If you are a 'fussy' eater, aim to include any vegetables or fruit you like in every meal.

When you look at your meal plate, at least 1/3 should be covered by vegetables or salad.

Aim for 5 to 7 portions a day (38).

A portion is

Vegetables and Salad

Fruit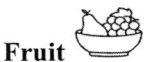

- *2 Broccoli spears*
- *4 tablespoons cooked Kale, spring greens or green bean*
- *3 heaped tablespoons of cooked vegetables such as carrots, peas or*

- **Small fruits** – 2 plums, 2 satsumas, 2 kiwi, 3 Apricots, 6 Lychees, 7 strawberries or 14 cherries.
- **Medium sized fruit** – 1 Apple, 1 banana, 1 pear, 1 orange, 1 nectarine, 1 peach.

- *sweetcorn or 8 cauliflower florets*
- *SALAD – 1 ½ full length celery sticks, 5cm piece cucumber, 1 medium tomato, 7 cherry tomatoes*
- *Tinned and frozen vegetables 3 heaped tablespoons*
- **Potatoes do not count as vegetables because they contain a lot of starch. All potatoes are included as starchy carbohydrates.*

- **Large fruit** – ½ grapefruit, 1 slice papaya, 1 slice melon (5cm wide), 1 large slice pineapple or 2 slices mango (95cm wide)
- **Dried fruit** – 30g or 1 heaped tablespoon, raisins, currants, sultanas, mixed fruit, 2 figs, 3 prunes, 1 heaped tablespoon banana chips.
- Canned fruit = 2 pear or peach halves, 6 Apricot halves, 8 segments of grapefruit or mandarins, 2 tablespoons of sliced fruit or mixed fruit.
- *Dried fruit contains sugar and is sticky so sticks to teeth. Fruit contains natural acid. Sugar and acid cause tooth decay. Eat as part of a meal, not in-between meals. Tooth decay is worse with repeated exposure to sweet, acidic foods or drinks that are sticky. Chewing releases saliva which contains bicarbonate. Bicarbonate helps neutralise the acid in food.

Fruit juice contains a lot of sugar particularly fructose which the human body does not process well in large amounts. If you want to drink fruit juices, a sensible compromise would be to have one glass a day, drunk with a meal. A 200ml glass of fresh orange juice contains the juice of about three oranges. Concentrated would contain the juice of four to five oranges. Eating three to five oranges in one go would be overeating, that's what you get in juice. It's easy to drink and terrible for your teeth because it contains both acid and sugar.

A 200ml glass of smoothie would be a better swap or buy favourite fruits and eat them whole such as strawberries, mango, raspberries or cherries.

Sometimes people are put off eating fruit because it needs peeling, or the juice is messy. Any fruit is good so buy a version that is neater to eat such as pre-prepared fruit salads or canned fruits or peel and slice.

Quality not quantity

Summary – Vegetables, salad and fruit

- It is widely accepted that fruit, vegetables and salad are beneficial to human health.
- It is known that in countries where the people eat between five to seven portions of fruit, vegetables and salad every day, the people living there have lower incidence of certain cancers, stroke, heart disease and dementia (diseases of aging).
- Not everyone likes vegetables, salad and fruit. Find ones that you do and include in your meals every day. Try more foods with hidden vegetables or fruit.
- If you eat a dessert, choose one that includes fruit or add fruit, such as fruit crumble, banana and custard, sliced fruit and ice cream.
- Frequently, children do not like the taste of vegetables because they have immature taste buds. When children become adults, taste buds become more sensitive to subtle flavours and texture, so they find more fruit and vegetables they enjoy.

Chapter 18

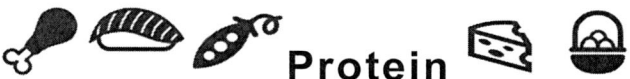 Protein

Literally every function in the human body is controlled by proteins. Protein in food is broken down by your gut into its building blocks, the amino acids. There are 22 different amino acids that your body uses to build new cells.

When people eat food, the body absorbs the protein it needs to maintain and build new cells. Any excess protein from the food is broken down and used as energy. Protein can be converted into glucose.

Protein takes longer than carbohydrate to digest, so the human body gets **energy from protein four to five hours after eating. Meals that contain about 1/3 protein rich foods slow down the rate of digestion. Makes you feel 'full' for longer and less hungry in-between meals.**

Most of the protein we eat is from the muscle of an animal or fish. Muscle tissue in any creature is mainly protein. All living cells have protein as part of their structure so all foods from plants contain some protein. The only foods that do not contain any form of protein such as, refined sugar, fats or oils are pure energy which has been taken out of a plant or animal.

If you do not eat meat, poultry, game or fish, you can get all the protein your body needs from different food combinations. Protein from animals (meat, poultry, game, fish, dairy foods) provide all the amino acids the human body needs. The protein in most plants has some but not all amino acids. The exception is soya which contains all the amino acids. Throughout history, people all over the world learnt that combining certain foods kept them healthy as well as giving them a satisfying meal that tasted good.

Food combinations that provide all the amino acids and work to lower the GI of a meal

---

1.   Pulses – beans, peas, lentils with dairy products (milk, cheese)
Baked beans with grated cheese. Dahl with natural yogurt.

---

2.   Wholegrains – brown rice, noodles, couscous,
Whole-wheat bread with pulses (beans, peas, lentils)
Baked beans on toast, risotto with peas, Mexican tortilla with refried beans

---

3.   Pulses (beans, peas, lentils) with seeds and nuts
Hummus (chickpeas with sesame seeds), mixed bean salad with flax seeds, vegetable and bean stir-fry with peanuts

---

4.   Dairy (milk, cheese) with wholegrain bread
Cheese sandwich with wholemeal bread, porridge with milk

Eating extra protein does not encourage muscle growth; only muscular exercise over time will build size and strength.

Protein helps to control appetite because it takes longer to digest, giving a slow release of energy.

Proteins are made up of complex building blocks that take longer for your gut to breakdown. This means any excess protein in a meal is used for energy about **four to five hours** after a person has finished eating. If someone ate two scrambled eggs on two toast for breakfast, their body would use the carbohydrate energy from the toast for about two hours then the protein would provide energy later. This has the effect of **controlling appetite (desire for food) or cravings (strong drive to eat) at the next meal**. The body is getting a slow flow of energy, so the brain does not need to drive overeating or choice of foods high in fat and sugar. This means people can eat less, feel energetic, make healthy food choices and feel satisfied with what they eat.

Do you struggle with feeling hungry?

It helps to reduce your carbohydrate portions to 1/4 of your meal plate or roughly 25% of what you eat. Swap for larger portions of protein foods, vegetables and salad.

Summary – Protein

❖ Foods high in protein included in balanced meals, snacks and desserts help to control your appetite.

Chapter 19
Fat

Fat is needed in our diets.

Eating fat does not make you fat. Fat is just the way that plants and all creatures including humans store energy.

What is fat for?

- ❖ **Energy** for movement, brain and body function.
- ❖ **Essential fatty acids** – the human body cannot make omega 3 and omega 6 fat from other fats we eat. So, we need to eat foods that contain omega fat.
- ❖ **Proper functioning of nerves and brain**.
  Every nerve in the human body is covered by myelin, a fatty material which wraps around nerve cells so they can send electrical messages.
- ❖ **Healthy skin**
  Produces oil to keep skin soft and supple. Skin is the barrier to protect the inside of our bodies. All cells in your body have a membrane (like wearing a coat) that is made of fat. This keeps fluid inside and outside the cell separate.
- ❖ **Transporting fat-soluble vitamins**
  A, D, E and K around the body to where they are needed.
- ❖ **Fats form steroid hormones**
  Steroids reduce inflammation.

Digestion

Once food is in the stomach being churned into soup, the fat does not mix well with water so collects at the top of the stomach. You can see this when you wash up a greasy pan the oil droplets float to the surface and collect together. This fat layer at the top of the stomach has an effect of making you feel full and satisfied which stops you eating. Plus, fat takes longer to digest than carbohydrate, so energy is released slower stopping you feeling hungry for a good four to six hours, or through the evening until the next day.

Fat is stored as triglyceride (34)

Fat is made up of **fatty acids**. The liver puts three fatty acids with one glycerol molecule, to make a triglyceride which is stored in a fat cell (adipose tissue). When our body releases stored body fat, it gets fatty acids to use as a fuel for movement, to generate heat and energy to drive body processes.

When fat is broken down, it produces waste products of water and carbon dioxide. The water is beneficial to the body and the carbon dioxide disappears as we breathe.

The liver can turn excess carbohydrates that are not used for energy into triglycerides (stored body fat). So even if someone ate a very low-fat diet, if they ate more calories than their body used up, it gets stored as fat. Fat is nature's way of storing concentrated energy.

Fat has been considered a 'bad' food since the 1960s

People often think that eating fat makes them fat. A common belief is that when a person eats fat, it deposits in their body especially around the abdomen (belly fat).

We only build up excess body fat when we habitually eat more calories than our body needs. It is the amount of food that people choose to eat every day that defines their body weight not whether the food is high in fat.

Healthy eating advice

Advice to cut down on fat began in 1958 after Ancel Keys, an American Physiologist, looked at statistics. He linked the fact that people living in countries who ate high fat diets had more heart attacks. Since then, **research has proved**

that heart attacks are not caused by eating too much fat; it is more complicated than that. There are many risk factors, high cholesterol is one, so is smoking, a family history of heart disease, an inactive lifestyle and obesity. The more risk factors you have and for longer, the greater chance of developing heart disease which is likely to cause a heart attack.

We now know (39, 40, 41, 42, 43)

Dietary fat is not the determinant of either high cholesterol or heart disease. Heart attacks, known as MI (Myocardial infarction) happen after a damaged artery wall gets clogged up with a mixture of cholesterol, calcium and fibre. This is how the human body seals up a damaged artery wall. The trouble is once the fat plug is there, overtime more cholesterol sticks to it and builds up, which gradually fills up the space in your artery. This reduces the blood flow to the heart and makes it more likely a blood clot will form and block the vessel (heart attack). Once an artery on your heart is blocked, your heart is deprived of oxygen and nutrients and it starts to fail. The amount of damage to your heart depends on which coronary artery is blocked.

The **Lyon diet study** (44)

Compared people who ate a **Mediterranean diet** (low GI carbs, lots of fruit and vegetables, olive oil) to **western diet** high in saturated fat, sugar and refined high GI starchy carbohydrates. The study concluded that Western diets increase the amount of **triglyceride** (fat that can be made from excess sugar and high GI carbohydrate). **High triglyceride is linked with increased inflammation which damages cells. This makes medical conditions characterised by inflammation more likely to happen.**

Research so far has proved that liquid fats such as olive, fish oils are beneficial to our health. Especially those rich in omega 3.

Beneficial Fat

Stick to natural solid or liquid fats; butter, coconut and liquid vegetable, nut, seed or olive oils. Oily fish is a very rich source of omega 3 and omega 6 essential fats that the human body needs.

Reminder – fat is nature's way of providing concentrated energy. So, make sure you have an idea of the calories you are eating to be able to plan meals and make choices of ready-made foods that meet what you need (calories).

Remember – it's eating habits that determine your weight.
The amount and choice of foods you habitually eat every day.
It is recommended to have two portions of fat added to a meal. No added fat needed if the foods you choose are naturally high in fat (oily fish, cheese, any fried foods, nuts, seeds, coconut). Some meals people choose to eat contain more fat than two portions, that's okay, just be aware of the calories you are eating, you may need a smaller serving.

It is better to spend your time gaining knowledge about the number of calories in foods than worrying about the amount of fat.

Examples of one portion of fat:

- ❖ 15ml or 1 tablespoon of liquid fat/oil **75 to 100kcals**
- ❖ Solid fat, butter, margarine, ghee, coconut
  1 teaspoon 5 to 6g = **55kcals**
- ❖ 1 tbsp full fat salad dressing or cream cheese
- ❖ 2 heaped teaspoons of mayonnaise
- ❖ Be aware of low-fat products. Check the ingredients; in many low-fat ready-made foods, the fat is replaced by sugar or glucose-fructose syrup or sweeteners or starches.
- ❖ Look at labels to see how many calories you will be eating.
- ❖ Low fat products may contain added sugar and because the fat has been removed, people miss out on the sensation of feeling 'satisfied or full' in the stomach. People are more likely to feel hungry again only one to two hours after a meal or snack. Even if the low-fat food was less calories, people are likely to eat more later in the day.

Be sensible with deep fried foods, these will push up the calorie content of your meal.

For example, the average portion of chip shop fish and chips is 1000 kcals a serving. Over half your calorie intake for one day in one meal *(average calories for people aged over 40)*. Pasties are high in fat, for example, the average calories in a Cornish pasty is 800, an individual 'full crust' pie is 500.

Summary – Fat

- ❖ Eating fat does not make you fat. It is the number of calories a person gets into the habit of eating every day that defines their body weight
- ❖ Fat should be included as part of a healthy meal. Fat is concentrated energy, so the more in a meal, the higher the calories
- ❖ Fat in a meal helps us feel satisfied and 'fuller' for longer
- ❖ Choose to eat natural fats that have not been changed by food processing or heated to high temperatures (frying)
- ❖ Omega 3 fats are beneficial to human health

Chapter 20
Energy

What do I need?

It's helpful to know the typical amount of calories, your body needs to function and for your lifestyle.

Once you know the average calories to maintain your current weight, you can plan how to reduce the amount you eat.

Reminder – A sensible reduction in your calories is wise rather than 'depriving' yourself by switching to a very restrictive diet. We now understand that dramatic changes to established eating habits do not last long.

Stored body fat is released if you eat less calories than you use up *(body function and movement)*

Structured eating with **low GI carbohydrate** and **balanced meals** will control your appetite; making it **easier to tolerate eating less** without feeling fatigued and avoiding episodes of overeating.

Fasting for twelve hours overnight makes the body switch to using more body fat for energy. Muscles will be protected because gradual weight loss is loss of fat not loss of body composition *(mix of water, muscle tissue and fat).*

Counting calories does not have to be perfect or exact. But having a rough idea is helpful.

Average daily calorie intake (45)

Age	Males	Females
0–3 months	550	500
3–6 months	600	550
7–12 months	750	700
1–3 years	1100	1000
4–6 years	1500	1500
7–10 years	1950	1900
11–14 years	2400	2300
15–18 years	3100	2500

As humans develop, they need more energy to keep the body functioning and to allow growth. It is interesting to see the increase in calories as children grow, with the largest food intake needed during adolescence for 'puberty'. Puberty is the rapid growth spurt developing from a child to an adult body shape.

Adults	Males	Females
19–34 years	2750	2200
35–64 years	2600	2100
60–64 years	2400	1900
65–74 years	2350	1900
75+ years	2300	1800

UK Energy Requirements based on the average energy required for people of a healthy weight who are moderately active.

You can see that boys and men, on average, need more calories than women. This is linked to males having more muscle than women. The more muscle you have, the more energy the body uses up in everyday life.

After the age of sixty, people need a bit less energy (food) to maintain their weight. This is linked to a gradual slowing of the rate an older body uses up energy (metabolism). Older people lose muscle mass and gain more body fat, this is made worse if they find it difficult to keep active.

Follow this plan

1. Work out your average daily calorie requirement on a calculator

2. Reduce the number of calories by 500

3. Plan a calorie range for each meal

Start looking at and working out the calorie content of meals, snacks and desserts and drinks you choose the most often…

Easy information – look at packets, search on the internet, consider getting an app that will tell you the calorie content of different foods. Look on websites, such as, BBC Goodfood (47) – gives nutrition information and calorie content of popular meals.

Round the calories to sensible number, does not have to be perfect or exact.

It is crucial to be patient with weight loss. Losing fat means you may only see small weight changes and if you are including exercise body weight is likely to increase in the short term due to an increase in muscle mass.

Remember these changes are improving the health of your body, do not give up.

Use the equation below to work out your average calorie intake (46)

OR download an app that will calculate this for you

Adult Males		Adult Females	
18–30 years	16.0 X weight in kg + 545	18–30 years	13.1 X Weight in kg + 558
30–60 years	14.2 X weight in kg + 593	30–60 years	9.74 X weight in kg + 694
60+ years	13.5 X weight in kg + 514	60+ years	10.1 X weight in kg + 569

The number calculated is the **BMR or basal metabolic rate**; this is roughly the **calories needed for your body to function NOT** for any activity.

If you want 'fast weight loss' and have in the past tolerated very restrictive eating, less than 1000 kcals a day, it would be wise to aim to eat the minimum calories your body needs to function (BMR). Otherwise within a few weeks, your metabolism (rate of calorie burning) drops. Back into the vicious cycle of tired, with food cravings.

Next, consider how active your lifestyle is.

Physical activity

The body needs energy from food for movement and clear thinking
Energy expenditure = **BMR** X Physical activity level (**PAL**) (48)

PAL is a way to express a person's daily physical activity as a number

Lifestyle	Description	PAL (49)
Sedentary	**Little to no activity** sit for majority of the day. Unable or unwilling to exercise. Limited mobility	**1.2 Women and Men**
Light Activity	Move around some of the day, **standing and walking for 1 to 2 hours.** Spend a lot of the day sitting	**1.4 women** **1.5 Men**
Moderate Activity	**On feet for most of the day, standing and moving about.** **Examples,** working in a shop Or works sitting at a desk but is active for one to two hours a day (walking to work or dog walking or exercise)	**1.6 women** **1.7 Men**
Very Active	**Hard daily activity** – physical labour – heart rate increases, feel hot, sweat **OR** work long day on feet, walking around with lifting and moving objects, examples, factory worker, builder, healthcare worker, farm work or gardener	**1.8 women** **1.9 Men**
Highly active or strenuous work	**Significant amounts of sport or strenuous work or leisure activity** *Example*: Competitive cyclist	**2.0 Women and men** ❖ **2.4**

Energy needed for body function (BMR) multiplied by the PAL can be used to calculate the amount of food energy (calories) a person needs for their typical lifestyle.

First example:

A man aged 56 works in an office, sits at a desk most of the day, uses a computer and phone. Travels by train has 30-minute brisk walk to and from the station 5 days a week. Plays golf all afternoon one day at the weekend.

- Activity factor = **1.4 Light Activity**

122

- **Weight** = 14 stone 8 lb or 92.5kg
- **Height** 5 foot 11 inches or 180cm
- BMI 28.5 – overweight range

14.2 X 92.5 + 593 = 1906.5
Round to a sensible number 1900.
Then 1900 X 1.4 = 2660
*Round to nearest 50 = **2650** total average calories a day*.
People do not eat food to an exact number of calories. Round up your calculation to the nearest 50 or 100.

A calorie range is more helpful than trying to eat to an exact number. It is impossible to eat to a set number of calories and gives the impression of either over or undereating.
To gradually lose fat, take 500 kcals off your total average calories

For this person to lose fat, he should aim to eat 2150 calories a day.
It is difficult to eat to an exact number so allow an extra 200kcals on top. This gives a bit if flexibility if you eat a bit extra or misjudge the calorie content.
Aim to eat daily calorie range between 2150 to 2350 calories a day

2nd Example:

Female aged 45 works part time in a shop. Has teenage children and a dog. She is the primary carer for her children and housekeeper because her partner works long hours.
Walks dog most days for 30–45 minutes.

- **Moderate Activity level 1.6**
- **Weight** 11 stone 2 lb or 70.8kg
- **Height** 5 foot 6" or 168cm
- **BMI 25** – beginning of overweight

9.74 X 70.8 + 694 = 1383.59
Round up to the nearest 50 or 100 = **1400kcal**
Then 1400 X 1.6 = 2240
Round to the nearest 50 = **2250 kcals a day**

To gradually lose weight *(take 500 calories off total with flexible 200 calories on top),* **aim to eat daily calorie range between 1750 to 1950**
(see example meal plan with calorie ranges on page 98)

Do you feel put off by equations or numbers?
Don't want to do any maths?

There are apps that will do this for you

All you need is your age, height and weight and the app will calculate your average calorie requirement to maintain your current weight.

1. **Know how many calories you need to lose weight**
2. **Plan the best times to eat meals and snacks**
3. **Do your best to stick to flexible calorie ranges**

Think about the demands of your day and **plan time windows** when you are most likely to be able to eat. **Divide your daily calories up to sensible amounts** that reflect the amount of food you would eat. Breakfast is likely to be the smallest meal, then midday meal and evening meal as the largest of your day.

Do not be put off by the numbers they are a practical way to compare what your body needs with what you are actually eating. **Start looking at how many calories are in the foods you eat the most often.**

Be aware of the energy your body needs. If you are busy, forget or unable to eat in your time window, eat as soon as you can or add the calories onto your next meal. Do not leave food until late afternoon or evening this is **the restrict overeat pattern** of eating.

Meal Plan (for example no. 2) with flexible calorie range

Meal/Snack	Time Window	Calorie range	Total Calories
Breakfast	7.00–7.30	200–250	900–975
Morning snack	9.30–10.00	100–125	
Lunch	12.30–13.30	550–600	
Mid-afternoon	15.50–16.00	100–125	900–975
Dinner	17.30–18.30	800–850	

Average daily calorie range to lose body fat = 1750–1950

Time windows are important to keep an ordered eating pattern. As long as you have purchased or prepared your meal and have started eating within the window, it will work.

Sometimes you will need to eat even if you do not feel hungry, especially in the morning.

Hunger catches up with you. What you eat in the morning will control your appetite in the evening.

Snacks may be needed to control hunger, so you do not feel a strong drive to eat at the next meal. If you are 'craving' food, you will eat more than you planned or be left feeling unsatisfied or deprived.

A flexible 200-calorie range is helpful because if you try to stick to an exact number, you may try to eat under it becoming too restrictive. Also, people may feel they have failed if they eat over their calorie target.

Eating at the top end of the range is for the days when people feel tired and hungry have been more active or are offered extra food. It allows us to eat a bit extra unplanned food. Sometimes people change their mind, desiring food that is higher in calories.

What if you keep eating more than the calories for weight loss?

Try fasting for 18 hours eating only two balanced meals, no desserts, no snacks, within a six-hour period; three to four days in a week?

- After fasting for 18-hours, go back to 12-hour overnight fasting. Aim to eat the calories needed to maintain your weight not the calories to lose weight on the 12-hour fasting days.
- **Use the 18-hour fasting days as the time to lose fat.**

Social eating, special events and holidays

Usually involve access to larger and higher calorie meals. Either eat your total calories for the morning at lunch or total calories for the afternoon and evening at dinner. It means do not eat snacks and aim for the top end of your calorie range. Otherwise, forget fat loss for one day and allow yourself full weight maintenance calories.

It does not take long to be able to make a reasonable estimate of the calories in food. A lot of what we like to eat we eat often.

The effort put into understanding the calorie content of different foods will make it easier for you in the future.

Eat and repeat – know the calories in foods you enjoy and eat most often.

Summary – Energy

- ❖ **People do not follow 'dieting' advice long term.**
- ❖ **Workout how much energy (calories) your body needs to maintain your current weight. Take off 500 calories.**
- ❖ **Gain personal experience with a new pattern of eating.**
- ❖ **Discover how many calories are in the foods you choose to eat the most often.**
- ❖ **Find out what works best for you.**

Chapter 21
Portions

How much should I eat? (37, 50, 51)

For meals that you prepare, there are different options.
Decide which would help you.

Simplest

Judging and serving a balanced meal just by eyesight
Based on using a standard sized dinner plate: measured 10–12 inches or 25–30cm diameter.

- Do not serve food in layers or pile foods on top of one another.
- It helps to serve 'neat' meals where the different food groups can be seen clearly.
- Once the meal is served, you can mix it up to combine flavours.

1. Serve starchy carbohydrate on **no more than 1/3** of your plate.
2. Serve the food high in protein on **1/3 of plate.**
3. Vegetables or salad (generous serving) **1/3 of plate.**
4. Fat one to two portions added as part of meal or in food naturally or as a gravy or sauce or added during cooking.

Look at the calorie content of foods you buy. Pre-package foods should have the calories written on the packet.

If you are making a meal by following a recipe and it does not tell you the calorie content, have a look on a website that offers recipes with nutrition information; the BBC good food is one useful website. If you decide to buy a cookbook, it helps to choose one that tells you the calories of each meal serving.

Get **a rough idea how many calories are in a snack or meal;** it does not have to be a perfect number. If you make a meal and do not know what is in it, then go on a website that gives nutrition information and search a similar version of the meal you are making.

If you weigh out foods, it's easy to search online or get an app that tells you the calorie content. Then put this portion into a measuring jug or a cup and mark or write down the measurement. This way, you won't have to keep weighing out your portions just fill the jug or cup to the level.

Are you thinking this is too much fuss and effort, I know I won't do that! People repeat eating the same meals and foods multiple times. Therefore, the effort you put into gaining knowledge about the calorie content will not need to be repeated again. Write it down or put into notes on your phone.

As part of my job as a dietitian, I would do calorie estimates in my head from someone's record of what they ate. It does not take long before you can make a reasonable judgement. Many of the people I helped had established knowledge of the calories in foods because they had spent so much time thinking about food when they were trying to lose weight.

Consider buying a portion control tool

Have a look on-line at:

➤ Portion plate
➤ 6-piece plastic portion set

➤ Three compartment food containers (great for preparing in advance to take to work or college or ready for when you get home).
➤ Portions Master

Portion control tools are a straightforward way to control the amount you eat by filling up the compartments, so you do not have to weigh out or measure.

Layered food that combines two or three food groups in a serving, such as cottage pie, lasagne, tortilla, should only fill 1/3 of a plate or one portion compartment.

Habits are established after about three months repeating new behaviours. That means it takes a lot of effort in planning and preparing what you are going to eat to establish healthy eating behaviours. **It will get easier with time.** A habit is something we do without thinking, feels automatic.

 **Reminder**

❖ If you eat meals at similar times each day, this gives your body the nutrients it needs to function well.
❖ This satisfies hunger, the body's need for regular energy.
❖ A consistent eating routine stops your brain driving your appetite (desire to eat) **so you will be able to tolerate eating smaller portions and make healthier choices.**

If switching to healthier foods is not working out:
That is, you do not enjoy the taste and do not feel satisfied after eating. Consider eating what you enjoy but controlling the portions. You will need to find out roughly how many calories there are in your favourite foods and limit what you eat to meet the calorie range planned for each meal.

If you like to feel 'full after eating':
Especially your main meal. Eat more vegetables or salad and add more protein foods; lean meat, poultry, game, fish, peas, beans, lentils, quorn, tofu.

If you don't like cooking or feel 'tired' and lack motivation:
Particularly at the end of the day, buy ready meals. Look for ones that are balanced, containing starchy carbohydrates, protein, fat and vegetables or salad.

Plus, the calorie content of the meal should be printed on the packaging, so you know how much energy you are eating.

When you have time, cook a meal once or twice a week that serves four to six people.

Portion according to the number of servings for the recipe and put in individual containers, chill or freeze. Build up a stock of home cooked ready meals.

Ideas for Low GI Breakfasts

50g or ½ cup (125ml) Porridge Whole Oats with 1 heaped dessertspoon of chopped nuts and 2 heaped dessertspoons chopped apple or berries + 200ml milk

Granola 50g + 125g natural full fat yogurt

Muesli 50g (no added sugar) with 200ml milk or 125g full fat natural yogurt

Homemade smoothies with 1 tablespoon of berries, 1 apple with 125g full fat natural yogurt and 1 heaped teaspoon of cinnamon

Quinoa porridge 50g with 1. Chopped apple and sprinkle of cinnamon

1 thick cut bread or 1 ½ medium bread or 2 thin slices of bread
(oatmeal or oat bran or granary or seeded or nut or soda)
With 2 heaped dessertspoons of peanut butter or any nut butter
OR/2 poached or scrambled eggs with butter
OR/2 bacon with 1 scrambled or fried egg with large grilled tomato or ½ tin of tomatoes
OR/1 poached egg with ½ small avocado
OR/2 heaped dessertspoons of cream cheese with pineapple ring or sliced tomato
OR/fried mushrooms, chopped onion and sliced tomato
OR/2 meat or quorn or vegetable sausages with tomato sauce
OR/2 large tomatoes sliced with 2 thick slices of mozzarella

2 egg omelettes with mushrooms, spinach, tomato and 30g grated cheese

1 Oatibix and 200ml milk or 125g full fat yogurt with 1 heaped dessertspoon of chopped nuts and 2 heaped dessertspoons of chopped fruit

Individual full fat pot of yogurt 125g with 1 large fruit sliced or ½ tinned fruit

Write a list of 'simple' meals that are easy to prepare and stick it on the fridge door

This helps for those times when a helpful prompt to decide on a quick balanced meal stops a person snacking.

Note: Milk and yogurts can be cows/Soya/Coconut

Ideas for simple 'quick' meals

Cooked fish fillet or tinned fish with large mixed salad + 1 heaped dessertspoon of full fat mayonnaise with four small or two large oat or seeded crackers

1 thick cut slice of granary, seeded or oat bran bread with 1 egg and ½ tin baked beans + side salad

1 burger bun sized granary roll with lean ham or quorn slices and 30 g grated cheese melted + side salad

2 thin slices of granary or seeded bread toasted with generous filling of ham, or beef, or chicken, or turkey or tuna or salmon or egg or houmous or vegetable pate optional mayonnaise or salad cream or mustard + salad in sandwich or on side

2 egg omelettes with any added mushrooms, peppers, sprinkle of grated Cheese 20g, etc. + 1 slice low GI bread + side salad

Small to medium sized jacket potato (size of your clenched fist) + tin of tuna and 1 heaped tablespoon of sweetcorn or 200g cottage cheese and pineapple chunks or chopped spring onions + side salad

1 tin of pilchards or sardines in tomato sauce on 1 thick cut buttered toast + side salad

1 buttered granary or seeded roll + 1 bowl of thick vegetable/tomato/meat/chicken/lentil soup (tinned or homemade) + sprinkle of grated cheese on top

1 large pitta bread with hot filling of fried onions with sliced steak or chicken or vegetable sausages + salad, full fat mayonnaise, mustard or chilli sauces optional

Ideas for side salad to fill side dish or side plate or 1/3 of your dinner plate

Mixed leaves of lettuce, cucumber, tomato, spring onions, watercress, etc.
Optional add 2 dessertspoons of sliced or tinned fruit e.g. pineapple or apple + 1 spoonful of nuts.
Or/1 heaped tablespoon of tinned sweetcorn, kidney beans or chickpeas.
Or/1 heaped dessertspoon of dried fruit or ½ a sliced avocado.
Or/olive oil and balsamic vinegar dressing or any oil-based favourite salad dressing 2–3 level tablespoons 30–45ml.
OR/ready-made bag of mixed salad from supermarket or salad selected from salad bar in supermarket.

Optional sauces – Mustard, salad cream, mayonnaise, chilli sauces, tomato ketchup or
dips e.g. tzatziki, hummus, salsa, taramasalata, guacamole

Ideas for low GI snacks between 100 to 150kcals
A small handful 30g nuts – salted, plain or dry roasted OR A hard-boiled egg
A piece of fruit – ½ grapefruit, 1 apple, 1 peach, 1 orange, ½ large banana, ½ mango, ½ pineapple with 15g nuts or seeds or coconut
½ Individual packet of peanut M&Ms 20–25g OR ½ individual tube of smarties 16 sweets OR Small white chocolate milky bar OR 1–2 individual dark chocolate with mint crème centres OR 2–3 squares of dark chocolate 25–30g
1 apple sliced with 2 teaspoons of nut OR peanut butter

2 Oat crackers with 2 heaped teaspoons of cream cheese OR full fat hummus OR peanut butter OR nut butter

Small individual bar of chocolate with high % of cocoa solids >50% or 30g chocolate covered nuts or 30g dark chocolate covered dried fruit

200ml flavoured soya milk drink OR 200ml drinking yogurt OR probiotic plain yogurt drink
Small or medium latte or glass of soya milk

Protein cereal bar or low carb cereal bar – look for carbohydrate content less than 15g per bar OR chocolate covered wafer biscuit

1 scoop of full fat ice cream – *size of ½ tennis ball to fit on top of wafer cone*
1 individual pot of crème caramel or a mousse (any flavour)

4 cherry tomatoes with 20g cheese – *size of 4 sugar cubes*

Individual packet of salted OR plain popcorn

1 scoop of diary ice cream or dairy free ice cream with 20g chocolate covered nuts or 1 sweet oat biscuit crumbled on top

1 large or 2 small sweet biscuits made with oats

Small banana sliced or ½ mango or 2 pineapple rings with 125g full fat yogurt/soya yogurt OR 1 scoop of ice cream (plain, no sugar syrup or chocolate pieces) OR custard

Individual tub OR 125g of full fat natural yogurt or soya yogurt OR custard with 1 heaped teaspoon of jam OR honey or maple syrup and sprinkle of chopped nuts or seeds on top

Summary – Portions

- ❖ It helps if you have different ways of judging the amount to eat for different situations.

  Have a look at websites that offer helpful, easy information on portion sizes:

  www.nutrition.org.uk. British Nutrition foundation. Find your balance – full portion size list.pdf

  www.bda.uk.com. BDA. The Association of UK Dietitians. Portion sizes: Food fact sheet.

  www.nhs.uk. NHS. The Eatwell Guide.
- ❖ Measuring or portion compartments can be used at home or for a packed lunch or picnics or whilst travelling.
- ❖ If you buy food at work or eat out, judge by eyesight and practice serving or ordering a balanced meal.
- ❖ All this gets easier with time. It is a lot of mental effort for three to four months after that new ways of eating are becoming established habits so there is less thought involved. People start to choose foods and eat amounts automatically.
- ❖ People rarely follow meal plans or recipes written by someone else long term. People adapt meals to a version they prefer.

Start planning your own simple meals and snacks.

Get a dry wipe or blackboard in your kitchen or on the fridge door and write down balanced low GI meals/snacks that you enjoy and are easy to prepare.

Use it as a shopping list.

Chapter 22
Social Eating

Everyone eats food. Families, friends and food contribute to a person's physical and mental wellbeing.

Food structures people's lives, provides social activity, defines relationships and represents ethnic identities.

A lot of time is spent planning and shopping for food to feed family, friends and partners. The food prepared and shared with others is one way to show that we care about them.

Holidays, festivals, religious celebrations, birthdays, eating in restaurants are defined by the expectation that there will be lots of food. People may abandon normal restraint during these events and end up eating large high calorie meals with several courses.

If people drink alcohol, there can be an expectation of drinking as much as you want. A person may feel a loss of control or a need to 'let go' with a desire to feel good and get pleasure from eating or alcohol.

If I am socialising, what do I eat?

Think about your eating habits.

How many courses would you eat?

Do you have side dishes?

Do you drink alcohol?

Do you care less about what you eat when eating out or on holiday?

Do you eat more if you drink alcohol?

Do you leave the restaurant feeling uncomfortably full?

If an advert for an all-inclusive holiday said…

 **Travel to beautiful countries**

Great entertainment

Luxury accommodation

Opportunity to binge on alcohol and food for two weeks

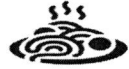 **Guaranteed weight gain**

Will have suntan, higher cholesterol and increase in blood pressure

---

No travel company would agree with this because no one forces us to overeat or binge on alcohol.

Overeating and binge drinking alcohol actually harms our health, but because the effects aren't immediate, we soon forget how rough it made us feel and then repeat the same behaviour.

Do your best to control what you eat and drink

Most people want to be fit and healthy. Practise turning your thoughts from short-term pleasure to thinking how great you will feel when you are slimmer and fitter. It helps if you remember a time in your life when you weighed less and were more active. If you have a photograph of yourself at a lower weight, put it somewhere like the fridge door as a motivator.

Making healthier choices is an important part of being kind to yourself. This means not behaving in a way that harms you.

Treat yourself like you would someone you are responsible for helping.

Another popular eating event in the UK is going for an Indian or Chinese restaurant meal or takeaway. Chinese and Indian cuisine offers a wide variety of meals with different flavours. Somehow, it has become normal to order excessive amounts of food.

For a typical Indian restaurant meal or takeaway, its estimated people eat about 1500kcals. This includes one main dish, a rice or whole naan bread and a side dish and a poppadum with sauces.

If people eat all that plus a second side dish or a whole rice and a whole naan or chapatti to themselves, they are looking at around 2500 calories for one meal, none of this includes the alcohol.

My point is **not** to be saying do not eat Indian or Chinese food, because it is delicious. It's to emphasise the reality that what is accepted as normal is **actually overeating**.

I would recommend you have:

- One main dish or half portion of two dishes or one quarter of four dishes
- Share a rice and a naan with someone else
- Share a side dish
- Include side salad or vegetables (not in oil) to fill up your plate and create a balanced meal

This is still a high calorie meal around 1000kcals, but it is not binge eating. If you love Indian or Chinese or Thai food, consider eating out more often to have favourite dishes or try different flavours. Ordering less food and drink at two meals rather than eating a lot at one may not cost you much more money. **You will know you're eating habits are changing if you can leave the restaurant feeling satisfied rather than 'stuffed'.**

Alcohol and food

Try not to combine alcohol and food or limit it to one drink with a meal. Separate these social events. Appreciate the taste of a great meal in a restaurant one night without alcohol and then another time go for an alcoholic drink without eating. If you drink wine or beer with a meal, the alcohol works to relax you and feel less inhibited so may care less about overeating.

The Liver

It is the liver's job to get rid of alcohol at about one unit an hour. Alcohol in large amounts is poison to the body so the liver prioritises getting rid of it. One job of the liver is to release stored glucose into the bloodstream. If a person binge drinks, the liver is not able to release as much glucose because it is dealing with breaking down alcohol. This makes a person feel tired and hungry so more likely to eat larger meals or keep snacking. Ever noticed that if you have a hangover, you feel better after eating?

Eating Out

People often feel compelled to eat a lot if they are paying for their meal or someone else is paying. Especially restaurants that offer unlimited servings such as buffets or all-inclusive hotels or cruise ships.

There's nothing wrong with eating out but if you want to change your eating habits to lose fat and not gain weight again, then changes need to be every day.

This means committing to sticking to new eating habits for any special social event and any holidays.

Socialise more, eat and drink less

Plan Ahead

If you know which restaurant you are going to, spend 10 minutes online looking at the menu. It is easier to plan what to eat away from any social pressure. By the time you get to a restaurant, you will be hungry and more likely to over order. Some restaurants have the calories on their menu; this helps make healthier choices.

Do not cut down or avoid eating in preparation for a meal out. This is giving yourself permission to overeat. **Keep ordered eating to feel in control of your food choices**. If you go to the restaurant with a strong appetite, it will be harder to stop eating until you feel full.

Speak Up

If you are going with family or friends who enjoy eating several courses and drink alcohol freely, you could feel under pressure to fit in with their eating habits.

Either stick to what you planned to eat and be determined or use a reasonable excuse such as, my doctor/dietitian has told me I need to eat less or drink less alcohol and make healthy choices. If possible, speak to people before the meal so you can relax and not worry about people persuading you to eat or drink more.

Keep your eyes on your own plate

Focus on conversation rather than what others are eating. If you ordered a healthier meal choice, you may struggle with feelings of 'missing out' especially if a person you are eating with has ordered one of your favourite meals. The thing is you cannot control what other people eat. Comparing your meal with everyone else is an unhelpful habit.

Healthy social
eating habits

Only ever 2
courses

3 courses is too
much food

Eat less to spend less
so you can eat out
more often

Side dishes are a swap
for a starter or
dessert

One of your courses
should be a favourite
so you feel satisfied
and not deprived

Pick one course that
is higher in calories
the second course
should be smaller
and lower in calories

At least 1/3 of what
you eat should be
vegetables or salad

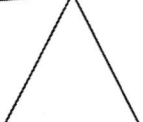

Summary – Social eating

❖ Practise new eating habits all day every day, this includes social eating
and holidays
❖ Plan ahead what you are going to eat and drink before going out, this
helps.

- ❖ Do not go to a restaurant feeling really hungry
- ❖ Quality not quantity
- ❖ Focus on the long-term goal of being healthy rather than short term pleasure gained from eating and drinking alcohol freely

Part 4

Chapter 23
Main Summary

How open minded are you to changing the way you eat?

Just imagine what life would be like if you lost fat, became more active and felt fitter

Do you feel willing to change?

Are you able to change?

Discuss the changes you want to make to eating and activity habits with partners and/or significant people in your life

Ask for their support

Change is a cycle that you need to repeat several times before your brain settles into new eating and activity behaviours

The experience of each cycle shows you what works and what does not

Lapses back to old eating habits are not a failure

Problem solve what went wrong and try again

What is the 'meaning and purpose' behind the desire to change eating and activity habits

Think about your patterns of behaviour that trigger

eating too much or bingeing on alcohol

The brain will keep driving you to maintain old behaviours

Change depends on understanding eating habits

TRIGGER – BEHAVIOUR – REWARD

THOUGHT – EFFORT – RESIST URGES

Food is not bad it's just energy

Get an idea how much energy (calories) is in the foods you choose to eat the most often

The human body functions at its best if it is given the nutrients it needs *(fat, carbohydrate, protein, vitamins, minerals, fibre)* in regular meals

If you deprive your body with disordered restrictive eating,

it will drive you to over eat or binge

Eat at similar times, even if you do not feel hungry

Stay in control of food choice and be in control of appetite

Structured, routine eating brings a sense of order

Fasting from **7 pm to 7 am** gives the human body

a break from dealing with food

Switches body to using more fat for energy

Helps to suppress your appetite during the day

For faster weight loss, 18-hour fasting. Eat 2 balanced meals *(no desserts, no snacks)* within a 6-hour period.

Aim to eat calories for weight loss *(calculate)*

Sugar is 'fast' energy, most people do not need it

Give it time, your taste buds will adapt

to prefer foods and drinks without added sugar

At least one third of every meal should be vegetables, salad or fruit	Choose low GI starchy carbohydrates as part of meals and snacks
Eating more vegetables, salad and fruit is a significant positive improvement to health	

You need to know roughly how many calories your body needs to hold its current weight, then take 500 calories off

Start looking how many calories are in foods you eat often and compare it to what you should be eating

When choosing a meal, think 'balance', one third starchy carbohydrate, one third food high in protein, one third vegetables or salad, one to two portions of fat

as part of or added onto a meal

If you struggle with feeling hungry,

increase the amount of protein and vegetables in your meals

Try different ways of 'quick and simple' portioning

Effort in the early days will be rewarded with knowledge about nutrition and healthy eating habits that are automatic

Take full responsibility for everything you eat and drink

Any regular exercise will improve your physical and mental health

Exercise improves body composition by using up stored body fat, building muscle and reducing insulin resistance

Dieting does not work long term because it only changes your body

Changing eating habits works because it transforms your body and your brain

Chapter 24
Health Boosting Changes

Priority order to 'kick start' your body into losing fat

What do I do first?

Week 1.

Overnight fasting

- No food or drinks that contain calories for twelve hours every day
- As often as possible, keep fasting between **seven in the evening** to **seven in the morning**

Week 2.

No fast carbohydrates

- No added sugar, no foods that sugar is listed as the first ingredient
- Definitely no sugar in drinks
- Swap the starchy carbohydrate foods you eat the most often for a lower GI alternative
- Reduce the amount of foods you eat made from white flour

Week 3.

Structured mealtimes

- Give your body what it needs to satisfy hunger (*physical need for energy*) and be in control of your appetite
- Eat at similar times; flexible half to one-hour time window to keep on track with your eating pattern

Week 4.
Balanced Meals

- When you look at the portions of food in your meal, it should be roughly one third starchy carbohydrate, one third vegetables, salad or fruit, one third a food high in protein and some fat added or as part of the food

Week 5.
Become more active

- Exercise will transform your body composition
- Gain muscle whilst gradually losing excess body fat
- Choose realistic exercise that will fit in around work and family life
- Choose exercises that make you feel good Mix them up

Week 6.
Swap the foods you eat the most often to healthier versions

- Increase the vegetable, salad and fruit content of your meals
- Quality not quantity
- Buy the best version of a food you can afford
- If meaning and purpose helps motivate healthy diet changes, consider free range or organic produce, vegetarian/vegan meals and more home cooking

Lifestyle change is hard work because your brain is 'wired' to repeat old habits

Commit to putting in time and effort every day for at least three months to establish new habits

Expect to lapse back into old habits as part of the cycle of change

As soon as possible *(ideally the next day)* repeat the new behaviours

Its not failure just experience

Give your brain time to adapt to different ways of eating and activity

Chapter 25
Guidelines

Start with number one, for a week, then keep changes moving forward by focusing on the next health boosting change each week. If after a few weeks one or more of these changes has stopped, then start back at the beginning. The repeat experience of the health boosting changes means you will be able to move through the stages quicker.

 Reminder

Change is a cycle that will need to be repeated several times before your brain allows new habits to replace the old.

If you feel impatient and want to see rapid weight loss, think about how long you have been overweight. How many times you have tried to 'diet' and ended up regaining all that was lost.

Establishing new eating and activity habits to permanently transform your body shape and health takes time.

Week 1
Get used to the overnight fasting for one week

- ❖ The fasting will switch your body to using more stored body fat for energy, plus it will help control your appetite during the day.
- ❖ After one-week, start cutting down on sugar (week 2)

Week 2.
Cut out added sugar and excessively sweet foods

❖ Cutting down on sugar lowers calories but most importantly, it stops rapid spikes in your blood glucose level.
❖ This has an effect of lowering insulin levels in blood, so your body spends less time storing energy and more time releasing; uses more body fat for energy during the daytime.
❖ When you have had one week getting used to life with less sugar, start eating at similar times each day (start week 3).

Week 3.
Eat at similar times each day

❖ This change is mentally demanding because you need to fit your life around your mealtimes rather than fitting food around your day.
❖ There will be a need to be selfish, putting your own needs above the demands of work or family.
❖ After one week of a more ridged eating routine, start paying attention to the balance and portion sizes of the foods on your plate (week 4).

Week 4.
Balanced meals digest slowly so control appetite.

❖ Putting more time into planning meals focuses attention on the nutrients you are giving your body.
❖ It is a way of increasing the amount of vegetables, salad and fruit in your diet.
❖ Spend ten minutes each day planning what you will eat. Good times for planning are either early morning or evening.
❖ Do not be spontaneous, thinking I will decide later what I am going to eat. It's easy to get distracted and once you feel hungry are more likely to go for convenient, ready-made, high calorie snack foods rather than a balanced meal.

❖ Make sure your fridge, freezer and cupboards are stocked with healthy low GI foods, so that when you feel tired and hungry, you will stick to new habits.

❖ It is more important to gain an idea of how many calories are in food rather than worrying about how much fat is in it.

On week 5, introduce physical exercise.

Week 5.

When you feel in control of your eating pattern and appetite, focus on being more active.

❖ If someone wants fast weight loss and chooses to eat a ve
❖ ry low-calorie diet and exercise, this is effective for about three months, then a combination of hunger and fatigue 'kick-in'. This is a trigger back to old eating habits and leaves people feeling less motivated, too tired to exercise, with a sense of 'whatever I do, I cannot lose weight'.

❖ To lose fat, work on changing eating habits first and then bring in exercise. Exercise together with dietary change is more successful in losing weight and keeping it off. Exercise on its own without dietary change has little long-term effect on weight loss.

❖ The human brain needs time to adapt to changes in eating routine, reduction in food portions and alcohol.

❖ Exercise will be easier at this stage because you will have lost some body fat, have more energy and feel less hungry

❖ Introduction of exercise maintains gradual loss of fat and promotes muscle development. Muscles are the big energy burning cells of the body. This starts the transformation to a more athletic body shape.

❖ Choose exercise you are physically able to do that fits around your lifestyle. Establish regular exercise sessions between thirty to sixty minutes, three to six times a week.

Week 6

Focus on healthier food choices.

Week 6.

At this point, you have a structured eating pattern and feel satisfied with smaller portions of a balanced meal.

Now is the time to start swapping the foods you eat the most often for a healthier version.

When people are stuck in a pattern of unhealthy food choices, healthy meals or snack choices are not as appealing. When eating is disordered, the body is not releasing enough stored energy, so people are driven to eat high calorie foods that are fast to digest. If you have adhered to the diet and activity changes in week one to five, then week six is a natural progression.

- ❖ Try different vegetables or fruits.
- ❖ Small servings of high-quality chocolate or cakes with high fruit and nut content (within calorie ranges).
- ❖ Eat less processed meat, poultry or fish, consider buying from a butcher or fishmonger who can advise you on the source and best cut.
  - ➤ Include more vegetarian or vegan meals.
- ❖ Rather than a carvery or 'all you can eat', consider a fine dining experience were flavour is more important than 'filling' portions.

At any stage, people may experience difficulties in their life which trigger old eating or alcohol habits. Demands from work or family or partners may need to take priority over exercising and healthy eating for a while.

Feel proud of yourself for what you achieved and the experience of great self-care. You will not forget it. Deal with what you have to and start planning to begin again at week one, overnight fasting, as soon as you can.

The experience of moving through all the stages means you will be able to establish changes faster than the first time. So, will be back on track in no time.

Chapter 26

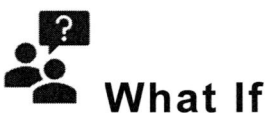 **What If**

What if I have a sedentary lifestyle?

Inactive, sit most of the day, minimal walking, either through choice or unable to be active due to a disability?

1. Weeks one to four and six *(overnight fasting, no fast carbohydrates, structured mealtimes, balanced meals, healthier food choices)* will make a significant improvement to health with gradual loss of excess body fat.

2. It helps to work out your average energy requirements and make a plan of calorie ranges for meals and snacks. Spend time learning roughly the calories in the portions of the foods you eat most often. Most people have no idea how many calories are in foods they enjoy; it is easy to eat more than you need.

3. As people age, body composition changes, losing muscle and gaining fat. Pay attention to your carbohydrate portions, you definitely **do not need fast carbohydrates** if your lifestyle is inactive. Go for **low GI starchy carbohydrates** and swap some of the portion for extra food rich in protein, vegetables, salad or fruit.

4. **When serving a meal cover one quarter of your plate with low GI starchy carbohydrate**, split the remaining plate, half vegetables or salad and half protein food.

5. See low GI simple meals for ideas on the portions and controlled portions of low GI carbohydrate.

If you need medication, check the side effects. Some drugs can increase appetite or increase insulin resistance, such as steroids and some anti-depressant medication. Do not stop taking any prescribed medication without discussing possible alternatives with a doctor first. Mental or physical health problems may take priority over the desire to lose weight.

What if I have type 2 diabetes?

Loss of body fat will lower insulin resistance. If a person with type 2 diabetes loses significant abdominal (belly) fat, they can reduce or stop needing medication or insulin injections to control their blood glucose level.

Diabetes and improving blood glucose control is all about losing excess belly fat.

Reducing the amount, a person eats and doing regular exercise achieves weight loss. Research (52) reports it does not matter if the diet is low in carbohydrates or low in fat, compliance is what works.

The trouble is old eating habits creep back in and people regain the weight they lost. Rather than low carb or low-fat diets, go for low GI carbs, control your portions, cut out fast carbohydrates. Be sensible with fat and go for healthy fats whenever possible.

1. **Definitely overnight fasting for twelve hours**, fourteen if you can manage it. To lose fat, control your appetite and improve blood glucose control.
2. **Definitely no fast carbohydrates, no sugar in drinks, no fruit juice, no sugary sweets.**
3. Focus on **controlled portions of low GI starchy carbohydrate with balanced meals**.
4. See Low GI simple balanced meals and snacks to get an idea of the mix and type of foods to eat.
5. **Any increase in activity helps lower insulin resistance**. The stabilising effect on your blood glucose lasts between 24 to 48 hours after exercise. To get rapid improvement in blood glucose control, incorporate six hours of exercise a week.

Follow health-boosting changes from week one to six.

If you have been prescribed medication, tablets or insulin to control blood glucose, as you start to reduce the amount of carbohydrate eaten, you won't need as much medication or insulin. Speak to your Diabetes Nurse or Doctor, so you feel confident to reduce these to prevent hypoglycaemia (drop in blood glucose below 3.5mmol/L).

Care for your body as well as you would look after someone you are responsible for.

What if I am very active?

What if I am overweight but have a physically demanding job or family life or do regular exercise?

People who have active lifestyles can find reducing what they eat difficult as they become hungry, tired and go back to go old habits in order to feel satisfied with what they eat.

1. **Definitely, overnight fasting will improve health and reduce body fat**.
2. Start with this and eat what you need to feel satisfied in the daytime.
3. Know your average energy requirements. Spend time looking at the calorie content of the foods you eat the most often.
4. **Focus on meal structure and balanced meals to control your appetite**.
5. If you do not eat breakfast, I would strongly recommend eating breakfast to gain control over what you eat in the evening.
6. Consider snacks between meals to take the edge off your hunger so you are able to reduce the amount eaten in the evening.
7. Increase the protein, vegetable/salad/fruit content of meals particularly at breakfast and lunch to stop snacking or second helpings later in the day.

 What if I am a fussy eater and hate vegetables?

Not everyone likes healthy eating. Some people do not like the taste of a lot of vegetables and salad.

1. **Definitely, the overnight twelve hours fasting**, to start losing fat and control appetite.
2. **Focus on structured mealtimes with controlled starchy carbohydrate portions**.
3. If you do not like the low GI or wholegrain starchy carbohydrates, such as seeded bread or brown rice, have a smaller portion of the one you like.
4. Include a snack between meals during the day to take the edge off your appetite before the next meal so you can tolerate a smaller portion. Another way is to spread food out, for example, take two rounds of sandwiches to work, eat ½ sandwich mid-morning, whole sandwich at lunch, ½ mid-afternoon. All this does is give your body energy slower over a longer time; it does not have to deal with a rapid surge in blood glucose from eating a big portion of high GI carbohydrates.
5. Try not to eat high GI carbohydrates on their own, such as white toast with jam, instead white toast with peanut butter or cream cheese or cheese on toast or scrambled eggs or meat, chicken or bacon sandwich.
6. Stop sugary drinks, give your taste buds time to adjust, for example swap sugar in coffee for a plain oat biscuit.
7. Even if you only like one or two vegetables or salad foods, include them in a meal as often as you can. Try meals where vegetables have been added and become part of the sauce such as stews or casseroles; disguises the texture and flavour.
8. Know your average energy requirements. Spend time looking at the calorie content of the foods you eat the most often. Compare the numbers to what you should be eating to lose weight.

 What if I binge eat?

Binge eating is having a sense of 'loss of control'. Everyone has random episodes of overeating. It's like the times we intended to eat two biscuits but end up eating half the packet or a few crisps or chocolates from the share bag then eat all of it while watching TV. Binges can be social and encouraged by others; all you can eat buffets, large three course meals with alcohol, restaurant meals or takeaways.

People who are unhappy about their body weight often have disordered eating which settles into a pattern of restricting what they eat around other people with secret or binge episodes when they are alone. The binges are driven by a combination of food cravings caused by food restriction and emotional triggers using food to distract or temporarily lift mood.

1. **Establishing a structured eating pattern is important**
   Set time windows to stick to a ridged eating pattern.
   This means committing to eating at times you do not feel hungry.

2. **Create an environment that does not make it easy to binge**
   Do not keep a large stock cupboard of foods. Stop buying foods you know you used to binge on.
   Speak to partners, family or friends and ask for their support.

3. **First focus on eating balanced meals at similar times each day**
   Then bring in overnight fasting from seven in the evening to seven in the morning.

4. **Allow yourself controlled portions of favourite foods that you used to binge on**
   Ideally, eat away from home because you are less likely to binge at work, with friends, family or in a restaurant or café.
   Do not buy food in bulk get one or two food items such as a chocolate bar and include it in your meal plan for that day.

5. **If eating out, plan a meal choice in advance**
   Order a meal in a restaurant before you have an alcoholic drink. Alcohol will lower inhibitions; you may care less about sticking to your meal plan especially if other people encourage you to eat and drink.
   Look up the menu online before you go out.

6. **Establish ordered eating**
   Wait until binge episodes are rare events or have stopped before you bring in exercise.

Ideally, start with exercise that is mainly muscular as it has a better effect on body composition (muscle gain) and does not make people feel so hungry.

Cardiovascular exercise such as running or cycling burns more calories but drives hunger so may drive episodes of bingeing.

7. **Lapses into binge eating is not a disaster**

Think about what was happening on the days leading up to a binge. Was it triggered by hunger or emotions? Look for behaviour patterns so you know when you are more likely to binge.

Distract yourself with something else which makes you feel good.

If eating has become disordered, get up the next day and start again with an ordered meal and snack routine.

Breakfast is extremely important to control appetite later in the day.

 ## What if I feel fatigued?

Fatigue is a feeling of extreme physical and mental tiredness. It's difficult to make changes to eating and activity habits if you have fatigue.

People who feel fatigued would be wise to focus on managing this before trying to lose weight. Are you getting enough sleep? Does your job or family life leave you feeling drained?

1. Structured eating with balanced meals and low GI starchy carbohydrates would help stabilise energy levels during the daytime.
2. No added sugar, sugary drinks or foods mainly made from sugar.
3. No caffeine after four in the afternoon.
4. Focus more on healthy food choices, more vegetables, salad and fruit, quality protein foods and fats; natural, unprocessed.
5. Exercise that would be the most beneficial is yoga or tai chi with or without meditation; muscular exercise that is mentally calming. When possible, exercise in the morning. Early activity lowers levels of stress hormones in the body and brain for the rest of the day; helps deal with anxiety.
6. Speak to partners, family, friends and ask for support.

Care for your body as well as you would look after someone you are responsible for.

What if I want to see fast weight loss?

Do you have a determined or impatient personality who decides 'I want to see fast weight loss'? Do you leave it until a few weeks before a holiday or social event to slim down to a weight you want to be?

It is possible to lose weight fast over a short period of time with low calorie diets, typically less than 1000kcals a day. This is not a lot of food.

Studies (56, 57) have followed people who have lost large amounts of weight found that the majority re-gain the weight.

Reminder – The history chapter explained how the human body copes with a starved state for about three months and then it drives you to eat to recover lost weight.

A pattern of yoyo dieting favours muscle loss as well as loss of body fat.

1. A **wise choice** for the impatient and determined would be too **fast for 18 hours** a day, eating two balanced meals within a 6-hour period. This works to switch your body to use mainly stored fat for energy. This suppresses appetite so people are better able to tolerate eating less calories. Aim to eat your weight loss calorie range within the 6-hour window to maintain healthy body function whilst losing body fat; stops the body going into starvation mode and slowing the rate, it burns calories.
2. Plan structured balanced meals with low GI starchy carbohydrates.
3. No added sugar, sugary drinks or foods with high sugar content.
4. For best results, exercise three to six times a week; aim for six hours exercise. Do weight training first followed by cardiovascular exercise. The weight training uses up glycogen stores (stored glucose) so the body has to release more body fat for energy during the cardiovascular exercise.

5. When you have had enough of 18-hour fasting, go back to 12-hour fast overnight, ideally 7 pm to 7 am in the morning; for maintenance of lost weight and to control appetite. You need to know your average energy requirements to plan what to eat to maintain your weight.

What if I love sweet foods, biscuits, cake, sweets?

I know I won't be able to stop eating them

Next time you go into a supermarket, bakers or corner shop spend a minute looking at the range of snacks, cakes and biscuits on offer. Food shops show you what the majority of people choose to eat. Each year, new products are introduced, if they don't sell enough, foods are taken off the shelves.

Not everyone likes healthy food choices. The main reason people become overweight is because of their eating habits; food choices and portion sizes. Habitually, eating more calories than their body uses up.

If you are thinking, I do not like healthy eating or low GI foods. That is your choice; no one can force you to eat foods you do not enjoy.

It is still possible to improve your health by losing body fat.

1. **Definitely do the twelve hours overnight fast**.
2. Structured meals and snacks. Plan time windows to eat and do your best to stick to it.
3. Know your average energy requirements. Start looking at the calories in the foods you eat the most often and compare it to what you need. Reduce portion sizes to meet your calorie range.
4. **Spread out your food** especially if they are made from high GI carbohydrates; white flour and sugar. For example, if you take a sandwich, packet of crisps and a chocolate bar to work. Eat the chocolate bar mid-morning as a snack, the sandwich for lunch and the crisps for an afternoon snack. This will control your appetite and reduce the surge in blood glucose simply by eating less at any one time. Commit to following an ordered meal and snack routine.
5. **Definitely eat breakfast** to control appetite later in the day.

6. Introduce exercise three or four times a week. Aim for six hours of exercise a week. Cardiovascular exercise suits people who eat high GI carbohydrates. Fast carbohydrates can be eaten around intense calorie burning activity such as running or cycling.

 ## What if when I eat more wholegrains, vegetables, salad and fruit, I get IBS?

IBS or irritable bowel is a common problem effecting the digestive system. Symptoms include bloating which may cause 'colicky' pain, alternating bowel habit typically constipation and/or diarrhoea. Healthy eating advice encourages people to eat more fibre because it helps control appetite by giving a 'full' sensation in the stomach and bowel which stops us eating too much. In populations where people regularly eat a lot of fibre, there is a lower incidence of bowel cancers.

Eating more gas-producing foods, like lentils, beans, cruciferous vegetables *(cauliflower, brussels sprouts, cabbage, bok choy, radish)* and increasing fibre intake with wholegrain breads or rice, doesn't suit everybody. Some people do not tolerate a high fibre intake.

Fibre is the part of plant foods that cannot be broken down by the human gut to use for energy so travels to the large bowel where it helps get rid of bowel waste by forming firm stools.

There are two types of fibre, insoluble and soluble. Insoluble fibre is known as 'roughage', like the bran in wholemeal bread. This fibre is the most likely to irritate the digestive tract. The second fibre is soluble, usually part of the flesh of vegetables and fruit. Soluble fibre easily dissolves in water and is broken down into a gel like substance in the bowel. This gel is helpful in preventing constipation and is much less likely to cause irritation or bloating in the digestive tract.

If when you eat more vegetables, salad and fruit you suffer with IBS, reduce the insoluble fibre content of your diet and see if this stops the bloating. Whole nuts and seeds can irritate some people's bowels. Rather than avoiding, try seeds or nuts that have been ground or turned into a smooth butter.

Ways to reduce insoluble fibre content of foods...

1. Take off the 'roughage' by peeling fruit and vegetables, such as apples, pears, carrots. The flesh contains beneficial soluble fibre.

2. Stop eating cereals that contain bran, such as bran flakes and mueslis. Swap for porridge, a granola or any cereal made from oats. Oats contain loads of soluble fibre.

3. Some vegetables, fruit, peas, beans or lentils cannot be peeled. Less likely to suffer with IBS symptoms if these have been cooked slowly for a long time in stews, casseroles or soups. This softens the fibre and makes it easier to digest. Canned vegetables or fruit are ideal because the canning process involves heating to a high temperature, making it digestible and non-irritant. Smoothies are blended whole fruit and/or vegetables. If you suffer with constipation, drinking a smoothie a day is a great natural laxative.

4. Stop eating wholemeal or whole grain bread and swap for a bread made from white flour with added oats. Some people get IBS symptoms after eating bread. They may be sensitive to gluten. Gluten is the protein part of wheat, rye, barley. If people are intolerant, it means the symptoms effect the bowel, rather than an allergy which effects the immune system, such as, coeliac disease. It is the protein part of foods that the body reacts too, so if a food is cooked, this starts to breakdown the protein and changes its shape or denatures it. The digestive tract is less likely to be sensitive to the food and react to it. So rather than excluding bread, try toasting it or choosing crackers or dry breads that have been cooked for a long time.

5. It's trial and error, you will learn which foods give you IBS and how much you can tolerate before symptoms start.

Chapter 27
References and Further Reading

(1). OED Online, Oxford University Press, June 2020
www.oed.com/viewdictionary

(2). https://www.nhs.uk

(3). Berkman, E.T. (2018). The neuroscience of goals and behaviour change: Lessons learned for consulting psychology. *Consulting Psychology Journal*, 70, 28–44.

(4). Aune, D., Giovannucci, E., Boffetta, P., Fadnes, L.T., Leum, N., Norat, T., Toustad, S. (2017). Fruit and vegetable intake and risk of cardiovascular disease, total caner and all-cause mortality: A systematic review and dose-response meta-analysis of prospective studies. *International Journal of Epidemiology,* 46 (3), 1029–1056.

(5) Centres for Disease Control and Prevention. (2014). Physical activity. Atlanta, GA: U.S. Department of Health and Human Services.

(6). Rebar, A.L., Elavsky, S., Maher, J.P., Doerksen, S.E., Conroy, D.E. (2014). Habits predict physical activity on days when intentions are weak. *Journal of Sport and Exercise Psychology,* 36 (2), 157–165.

(7). World Health Organisation. (2017). Global Health Observatory Data. Geneva, Switzerland: World Health Organisation.

(8). Rothman, A.J., Sheeran, P., Wood, W. (2009). Reflective and automatic processes in the initiation and maintenance of dietary change. *Annals of Behavioural Medicine, 38* (Suppl. 1), s4–s17.

(9). Verplanken, B., Wood, W. (2006). Interventions to break and create consumer habits. *Journal of Public Policy & Marketing,* 25 (1), 90–103.

(10). Van't Riet, J., Sijtsema, S. J., Dagevos, Hans., Jan De Bruijn, G. (2011). The importance of habits in eating behaviour. *Urban Economics, 57* (3), 585–596.

(11). Verplanken, B., & Orbell, S. (2003). Reflections on past behaviour: A self-report index of habit strength. *Journal of Applied Social Psychology, 33* (6), 1313–1330.

(12). British Nutrition Foundation. www.nutrition.org.uk

(13). Leading causes of death-office for National statistics. www.ons.gov.uk

(14). www.nhs.uk.Exercise

(15). https://www.gov.uk/government/publications/physical-activty-guidelines-infographics

(16). U.S. Department of Health & Human Services. President's Council on Sports, Fitness & Nutrition. Physical Activity Guidelines for Americans 2008. www.hhs.gov

(17). UK chief Medical Officers Physical Activity Guidelines. September 2019. assets.publishing.service.gov.uk

(18). Willis, L.H., Slentz, C.A., Kraus, E. (2012). Effects of aerobic and/or resistance training on body mass and fat mass in overweight or obese adults. *Journal of Applied Physiology, 113* (12), 1831–1837.

(19). Preece, J. *A brief history of Human Behaviour*. Great Britain. Amazon. 2013.

(20). Chatzi, C., Zhang, Y., Hendricks, W., Chen, Y., Schell, E., Gooman, R., Westbrook, G. (2019). Exercise-induced enhancement of synaptic function triggered by the inverse BAR protein, Mtss1L. *elife, 8* (24), e45920.

(21). Warburton, D.E., Nicol, C.W., Bredin, S.S. (2006). Health benefits of physical activity: the evidence. *Canadian Medical Association Journal, 174* (6), 801–9.

(22). Prochaska, J., Di Clemente, C. (1983). Stages and processes of self-change of smoking: Toward an integrative model of change. *Journal of Consulting and Clinical Psychology, 51* (3), 390–395.

(23). Buxton, K., Wyse, J., Mercer, T. (1996). How applicable is the stages of change model to exercise behaviour? A review. *Health Education Journal, 55* (2), 239–256.

(24). Sheldon, W. H. (1940). The varieties of Human Physique (An introduction of Constitutional Psychology). Harper & Brother.

(25). Krauss, W.S. (1985). The Aging body. New York: Springer-Verlag.

(26). Berg, J.M., Tymoczko, J.L., Stryer, L. (2002). Biochemistry. Section 30.3. *Food intake and Starvation Induced Metabolic Changes.* 5th edition. New York: WH Freeman.

(27). Maclean, P.S., Blundell, J.E., Mennella, J.A. *et al.* (2017). Biological control of appetite: A daunting complexity. *Obesity,* Suppl 1: S8–S16. doi:10.1002/oby.21771.

(28). Hopkins, M., Blundell, J.E. (2018). Energy balance, body composition, sedentariness and appetite regulation: Pathways to obesity. *Clinical Science, 130* (18), 1615–1628. doi:10.1042/CS20160006.

(29). Longo, V. (2018). The Longevity Diet: Slow Aging, Fight Disease. Optimize Weight. London: Penguin.

(30). The Eatwell Guide. www.nhs.uk.

(31). Ashraf, R., Aamir, K…Ahmed, T. effects of garlic on dyslipidaemia in patients with type 2 diabetes mellitus. *J Ayub Medical College Abbottabad.*

(32). Hewlings, S.J., Kalman, D.S. (2017). Curcumin: A review of its effects on human health. *Foods, 6* (10), 92.

(33). Habib, S.m., Jaward-Ur-Rehman., Shah, M.R. (2020). Synthesis of Lactobionic Acid based Bola-amphiphytes and its supplication as Nano-carrier for Curcumin delivery to cancer cells cultures in-vitro. *Int J Pharm., 21*, 119897.

(34). Reinus, J.F., Simon, D. (2014). Gastro-intestinal Anatomy and *Phy*siology. The essential. Oxford: John Willey & Sons.

(35). What is the Glycaemic Index (GI)? www.nhs.uk

(36). Brand-Miller, J., Leeds, A. *The complete guide to GI values.*

(37). Eating a balanced diet. www.nhs.uk Eatwell

(38). Why 5 a day? www.nhs.uk

(39). Suri-Tarino, P.W., et al. (2010). Saturated fatty acids and risk of coronary heart disease: Modulation by replacement nutrients. *Curr Atheroscler Rep, 12* (6), p384–90.

(40). Hu, F.B. (2010). Are refined carbohydrates worse than saturated fat? *Am J Clin Nutr, 91* (6), p 1541–2.

(41). Jakobsen, M.U., et al. (2010). Intake of Carbohydrates compared with saturated fatty acids and risk of myocardial infarction: importance of the glycaemic index. *Am J Clin Nutr, 91* (6), 1764–8.

(42). Hu, F.B., et al., (1997). Dietary fat intake and the risk of coronary heart disease in women. *N Engl J Med, 337* (21), p. 1491–9.

(43). Ascherio, A., et al., (1996). Dietary fat and risk of coronary heart disease in men: Cohort follow up study in the United States. *BMJ, 313* (7049), 84–90.

(44). Kris-Etherton, P., Eckel, R.H., Howard, B.V., Sachiko, S., Bazzarre, T.L. (2001). Lyon Diet Heart Study. Benefits of a Mediterranean-style, national cholesterol education programme/American heart association step 1 dietary pattern on cardiovascular disease, *103*, 1823–1825.

(45). British Nutrition Foundation (2016). Nutrition requirements. Macronutrients – Energy, fat, carbohydrates and protein. Estimated Average energy requirements. www.nutrition.org.uk.

(46). Henry, C.J. (2005). Basal metabolic rate studies in humans: measurement and development of new equations. *Public Health Nutrition, 8,* 1133–1152.

(47). www.bbcgoodfood.com

(48). Total energy expenditure (TEE) and physical activity levels (PAL) in adults: double-labelled water data. *Energy and protein requirements, proceedings of an IDECG workshop.* United Nations University. 1994-11-04.

(49). Human energy requirements: energy requirement of Adults. *Report of a Joint FAO/WHO/UNU Expert Consultation.* Food and Agriculture Organisation of the United Nations, 2004.

(50). British Nutrition Foundation. Find your balance-full portion size list.pdf. www.nutrition.org.uk

(51). The association of UK Dietitians. Portion sizes: Food fact sheet. www.bda.uk.com BDA

(52). Lanham-New, S. A., Hill, T. R., Gallagher, A. M., Vorster, H. H. (2020). Introduction to Human Nutrition. 6.7 Obesity 125–129. The Nutrition Society Textbook. 3rd Edition. Oxford: Willey Blackwell.

(53). Brandhorst, S., Young Choi, I., Wei, M., et al., (2015). A periodic diet the Mimics fasting promotes Multi-system regeneration, enhanced cognitive performance and health span. *Cell Metabolism.* Jul 7; 22 (1); 86-99.

(54). Liangyou, R. (2014). Energy Metabolism in the Liver. *Compr Physiol.,* 1 (4), 177–197.

(55). De Cabo, R. Mattson, M. P. (2020). Effects of Intermittent Fasting on Health, Aging and Disease. *N Engl J Med,* 382–298.

(56). Hall, K. D., Kahan. S. (2018). Maintenance of lost weight and long-term management of obesity. *Med Clin North Am.,* 102 (1), 183–197.

(57). Wu, T., Gao, X., Chen, M., Dam, R. M. (2009). Long-term effectiveness of diet-plus exercise intervention vs. diet-only interventions for weight loss: a meta-analysis. *Obesity,* 10 (3), 313–323.